D1369751

10 Breakthrough Therapies for Parkinson's Disease

ENGLISH EDITION

Michael S Okun MD

⋅→═◉ ◉═←⋅

Dedication

To Leslie, Jack and Gracie with all my love and appreciation for your many years of unwavering support.

Introduction

"Every challenge you encounter in life is a fork in the road.
You have the choice to choose which way to go: backward,
forward, breakdown or breakthrough."

— Ifeanyi Enoch Onuoha

A BREAKTHROUGH IS defined as a sudden increase in knowledge, improvement in technique, or fundamental advancement in understanding. Often breakthroughs occur when a formidable obstacle is penetrated. Breakthroughs are heralded as major achievements and they pave the road to meaningful progress in any disease. I have spent my entire professional career focused on Parkinson's and related diseases. I have been blessed to spend much of my time taking care of patients, and I have evolved to understand the critical need for all those suffering to have access to information on breakthrough therapies. The point that I emphasize with my patients is that breakthrough ideas and therapies in Parkinson's disease stretch far beyond a single drug or stem cell. There is, in fact, a broader and more exciting picture and portfolio of breakthroughs spanning drug, cell, vaccine, device, genetics, care, and behavior. Patients and families with personal investments in Parkinson's disease should be informed and updated about all of the potential breakthrough therapies. The purpose of this book is to inform, educate, and to inspire Parkinson's disease patients, family members, as well as health care professionals and scientists. Together, we will journey toward better treatments -- and one day a cure.

In a decade where newspaper headlines have been dominated with gloomy economic forecasts, most experts agree that health care expenses are driving much of the world's current economic burden. Austerity measures, if applied to research into Parkinson's disease, could have terrible long-term effects. The downstream effects of cutting off research dollars will limit breakthrough therapies and will damage the world's economic infrastructure.

Ray Dorsey from the Johns Hopkins University constructed the first sobering weather forecast for Parkinson's disease. In the world's most populous nations, the number of Parkinson's sufferers will double to almost 30 million by the year 2030.1 As life expectancy increases, so too will the number of young and old Parkinson's patients. A worldwide economic burden will create a nasty storm. This storm will quickly overcome every occupied continent on the planet.

Stacey Kowal from IHS Global Inc. and her colleagues constructed an economic model of Parkinson's disease. The model was designed to estimate "disease prevalence, excess healthcare use, medical costs, and nonmedical costs" all by using the U.S. Census Bureau's 2010 to 2050 population data. This model allowed the researchers to estimate the current and projected burden of Parkinson's disease. The model predicted that the prevalence of Parkinson's disease would double by 2040. Further, these researchers estimated that in the U.S. we will spend $14 billion dollars a year on Parkinson's disease care. This number is 8.1 billion dollars more than we spend on an American citizen without the disease. Additionally, 6 billion dollars will be lost due to employment issues.2

Andy Siderowf and colleagues at the University of Pennsylvania's National Parkinson Foundation (NPF) Center of Excellence took another approach to constructing an economic model. The Penn investigators were interested in the "economic consequences of slower rates of Parkinson's progression." They used a technique called a Markov model and predicted the potential savings associated with slowing Parkinson's disease progression. Slowing progression by 20 percent saved the health care system $60,657 per patient. Stopping disease progression saved $442,429 per patient.3,4

It is now clear that the weather forecast will be predicting a future storm of Parkinson's disease cases. This storm will be accompanied by a downpour of large hospital bills and an insurmountable economic burden. The newly diagnosed Parkinson's disease cases, when added to the existing patients, will have a social and economic impact on all countries and cultures. One point that I continue to harp on with my colleagues is that breakthroughs do not automatically translate into drugs or devices. Breakthroughs include all of the know-how and research into Parkinson's disease that enhance the lives of everyone affected. We will need to expand our notion of breakthroughs, and we will need to harness this knowledge to reduce the burden of Parkinson's disease. It will be important that we advocate for a strategic investment from all nations of the world.5

One of the most common questions I receive from Parkinson's disease patients and families is "What will be the next breakthrough therapy?" Because of the complexity of the disease, each person possesses a different combination of bothersome symptoms. This complexity means that the answer to the next breakthrough therapy will vary patient to patient, and it could be a breakthrough in care as well as possibly a new device or drug. I have been monitoring the breakthroughs in the field for the last 10 years as the National Medical Director for the National Parkinson Foundation. We run the free international Ask the Doctor web-based forum, and the questions posted have helped us to keep an accurate pulse on the field. Additionally, my blog called "What's Hot in Parkinson's Disease" and my guest columns as the associate editor for the New England Journal of Medicine's Journal Watch have provided the material, insight and inspiration for this book. Collectively, these experiences have provided focus for the topics in this book and in some cases the actual physical material. Several chapters include topics I have covered before, and in these cases I have added and updated information.6 The current book is an effort to provide a comprehensive review of the most important breakthrough therapies for Parkinson's disease. Consequently, these topics overlap with the most asked questions by patients and caregivers.

The unexpected runaway success of my first book, "Parkinson's Treatment: 10 Secrets to a Happier Life," has provided hundreds of messages and an ocean of feedback from patients, families and researchers. The majority of comments I received on the first book were focused on the need to understand breakthrough therapies and approaches. My desire is that this book will fill a knowledge gap and will provide hope and valuable knowledge to those in the Parkinson's disease community.

Michael S. Okun, M.D.
Adelaide Lackner Professor of Neurology
University of Florida Health Center for Movement Disorders and Neurorestoration
National Medical Director, National Parkinson Foundation
Email: michaelokunmd@gmail.com
Twitter: @MichaelOkun
Website: http://parkinsonsecrets.com

CHAPTER 1

Disease Modifying Drugs and Biomarkers

"One thing is sure. We have to do something. We have to do the best we know how at the moment. If it doesn't turn out right, we can modify it as we go along."

—Franklin D. Roosevelt

THE APPROACHES FOR treatment of Parkinson's disease can be broadly classified into three categories: 1) Disease modifying (also referred to as neuroprotective), 2) Symptomatic and 3) Cure based strategies. To date, there has been little progress on an absolute cure. The Holy Grail among the current generation of Parkinson's disease researchers has been the development and testing of drugs that can arrest or meaningfully slow Parkinson's disease progression. John King has been quoted as saying, "Learn to pause, or nothing worthwhile will catch up to you." A universal theme among all Parkinson's disease patients is the yearning for a therapy that would pause this progressive degenerative disease.

Inosine

I have spoken to many colleagues who evaluate patients and who conduct research into a variety of neurological diseases. I am convinced that the Parkinson's disease patient is possibly the most sophisticated consumer of health care. Although I sometimes struggle to remember all of the specific facts about the practice of medicine, I do remember that increasing uric acid levels can lead to a gout attack. I was therefore somewhat surprised when a recent patient asked me, "Should I take the drug Inosine to raise my uric acid levels? It may possibly treat my Parkinson's disease, and I may be willing to accept an occasional attack of gout." Though my first instinct was to say no, I have learned to accept that Parkinson's disease patients are frequently one step ahead of me.

Over the last 20 years, Parkinson's disease researchers have sought to identify compounds that when ingested will slow disease progression. One unlikely candidate was an old drug called Inosine. Inosine acts to raise uric acid levels in the blood. People with higher uric acid blood levels seem to be at a lower risk for developing Parkinson's disease. The immediate problem with this approach is that raising uric acid may result in an emergency room visit for kidney stones or gout.

Inosine is thought to work within the brain as an antioxidant, an anti-inflammatory and potentially even as an immunomodulatory molecule. While the exact mechanism(s) of action for Inosine remains unknown, it is known that the main consequence of using Inosine is raising uric acid levels in the blood. The association of higher uric acid levels with a decreased risk of later development of Parkinson's disease led a Harvard researcher named Mike Schwarzschild to the drug Inosine.[7-10]

Mike, along with the Parkinson Study Group, decided it was worthwhile to conduct a study "to determine the safety and tolerability of Inosine and its ability to raise urate levels in blood and cerebrospinal fluid in individuals with early Parkinson's disease." It was named the Safety of Urate Elevation in PD (SURE-PD) study. The design was a randomized double-blind placebo-controlled protocol, and its primary goal was to examine safety and tolerability in Parkinson's disease patients. Randomization was performed so that participants would not be aware of whether they received Inosine or a placebo, and the raters were blinded. A blinded rater was not allowed to be aware of which drug a particular patient was taking. The study was conducted in 17 sites and included 75 men and women with early Parkinson's disease who had not yet begun treatment with a dopaminergic medication. The blood urate level had to be normal (less than 6 mg/dL). Study participants received either placebo pills, pills to mildly elevate blood urate levels or pills to moderately elevate blood urate levels. Serious adverse events were similar in the Inosine versus placebo pill groups. Three people in the Inosine group developed kidney stones, and none developed gout. Inosine was considered reasonably tolerated. The study revealed that inosine could raise blood and cerebrospinal fluid (brain) concentrations of urate. The investigators actually performed spinal taps to be sure the drug could travel successfully from the blood to the brain. The study set up a second and ongoing investigation which is aimed to determine if Inosine will slow Parkinson's disease progression.[7-10] Investigators are also interested in whether there is a gender effect for Inosine as the results seem better in men compared to women.

Should you take Inosine to raise your uric acid level if you have Parkinson's disease? I do not yet recommend its use to my patients. Most of the available data has examined the risk of development of Parkinson's disease and has not addressed already diagnosed Parkinson's disease. Additionally, to date, many potentially disease modifying compounds for Parkinson's disease have been shown ineffective. The current data only showed us that Inosine was reasonably safe and that it gets from the blood to the brain. Inosine has not yet been shown to have a meaningful symptomatic benefit. Though the results of the current study are promising, we are still a distance away from declaring Inosine as an effective neuroprotective agent for early stage Parkinson's disease patients.[11]

Isradipine

Recently, Tanya Simuni and colleagues at the National Parkinson Foundation Center of Excellence at Northwestern University in Chicago tested another drug, Isradipine, as a potential disease modifying approach for Parkinson's disease patients. The idea was coined by a colleague of Simuni's at Northwestern, Dr. James Surmeier, who showed that this class of medications could be neuroprotective in the animal model. Isradipine works by blocking calcium channels and has shown promise in protecting brain cells from dying in animal models of Parkinson's disease. Isradipine is available in the United States as a FDA approved pill for the treatment of hypertension.12-14

Simuni and colleagues tested people with very early Parkinson's disease who did not yet need medications. These patients were randomly administered different dosages of extended release Isradipine or alternatively given a placebo pill. There were 99 patients enrolled in this initial study called STEADY-PD. The results revealed that Isradipine was tolerated less at higher doses, but there was no difference in the symptomatic effect with any dosage. The most common adverse events were swelling in the legs and dizziness. Simuni and her colleagues determined that 10 mg of Isradipine a day was the best dosage for a future clinical trial. There is now a 23 million dollar National Institutes of Health study that has been designed to examine the possible beneficial and disease-modifying effects of Isradipine. We are hopefully awaiting the results of this study. 12-14

Pioglitazone

Similar to Isradipine, another drug called Pioglitazone, which has been used for diabetes, has been repurposed as a potential Parkinson's disease therapy. Patients have begun to frequent our Parkinson's clinic and ask for the diabetes drug. What is fascinating about this particular drug is that it acts on a structure called the mitochondria (the energy producing part of the cell). It also reduces inflammation. Both mitochondria and inflammation have been implicated in Parkinson's disease pathogenesis. A multi-center study of early Parkinson's disease has been conducted to assess Pioglitazone as a potential neuroprotective treatment. Investigators collected measures of thinking and mood as well blood and urine biomarkers (a biomarker has been widely defined by many scientists as a measurable substance in human or animal which indicates the presence of disease, infection, or an environmental exposure).15,16 The study is complete, and we are awaiting the results of the formal analysis. Preliminary data presented recently at the International Movement Disorders Society suggested that the drug may not be useful in treating Parkinson's disease. However, despite the findings, it is very inspiring to think that drugs already FDA approved for other indications like diabetes could be repurposed for Parkinson's disease.

Creatine and Coenzyme Q10

A few promising neuroprotective drugs have recently proven to be disappointments. A high-profile drug recently tested for this purpose was creatine. Creatine is sold as a nutritional supplement and frequently utilized by bodybuilders. Creatine likely has many effects, and most people agree it can help to build muscle mass.17 However, is also has an impact on mitochondria, the part of your cells that biologists think of as the power plant. This part of the cell is damaged in Parkinson's disease, so it is reasonable to think that drugs that may help the power plant may be helpful in this disease. Unfortunately, the large NIH Creatine study was terminated early because of the overwhelming likelihood the study would not show a beneficial effect.18-20 We tell patients that if you are taking creatine for your Parkinson's disease and you feel it is helping, you don't have to stop it. Christopher Hass at the University of Florida National Parkinson Foundation Center of Excellence has shown many beneficial effects of creatine in Parkinson's disease beyond the possibility of neuroprotection.

Similarly, Coenzyme Q10 was also thought to be a neuroprotective and also symptomatic therapy for Parkinson's disease. There were, however, conflicting small studies in the literature on the effects of Coenzyme Q10. Recently, the Parkinson Study Group put Coenzyme Q10 to the test and observed that it was neither an effective neuroprotective or symptomatic therapy at both low and high (2400mg/day) dose.21-24

Nilotinab and Other Novel Compounds

There has been a great interest in developing drug therapies that may have the potential to decrease the abnormal protein deposits present in the brain's of Parkinson's disease patients. Fernando Pagan at the National Parkinson Foundation Center of Excellence at Georgetown has been testing just such a therapy. The drug, called Nilotinib, has been used in chemotherapy, but has been repurposed for its potential to "alter the abnormal protein build up in Parkinson disease and Diffuse Lewey Body Disease patients." Fernando's trial, which is listed on clinicaltrials.gov, is primarily interested in determining if disease symptoms change, if there are changes in the protein in spinal fluid, and to determine whether inflammatory markers in the blood change after taking Nilotinib. His hope is that this approach could slow down or stop Parkinson's disease progression. The results of the first safety study should be available soon.

Phil LoGrasso at Scripps Research Institute in Jupiter Florida has been keying in on another approach to modify Parkinson's disease progression. LoGrasso's approach has been to focus on a class of enzymes called jun-N-terminal kinsases (JNK). These enzymes are important for brain cell survival and LoGrasso has been working with industry to develop a new drug to target them.

Anti-Malaria Drugs for Treatment of Parkinson's Disease?

A research team from Nanyang Technological University (NTU) in Singapore and from McLean Hospital and Harvard Medical School focused on a brain protein called Nurr1. The protein is important in development and maintenance of brain dopamine cells and it may protect the cells from inflammation and from dying. Previous to this research study there were not any drugs known to bind Nurr1. The team screened approximately 1000 already approved FDA compounds and discovered that two antimalaria drugs (chloroquine and amodiaquine) act at Nurr1. The team has tested the compounds successfully in rats and will soon be pursuing human trials. This is a great example of using technology to repurpose already existing drugs.

Could LRRK2 and PARKIN Gene Mutations Lead us to a Therapy?

Approximately 10% of Parkinson's disease cases have been associated with gene defects. These changes in the DNA have allowed researchers to hone in on the mechanisms that may be responsible for this devastating disease. Scientists around the world have become adept at preparing animal models of Parkinson's disease by using the observed changes in the DNA occurring in some human cases. Ted and Valina Dawson, a husband and wife team located at the National Parkinson Foundation Center of Excellence at Johns Hopkins recently published an important paper on how the most common genetic subtype of Parkinson's disease (LRRK2) leads to degeneration and to cell death.25

Mutations in the DNA of Parkinson's disease patients located in the leucine-rich repeat kinase 2 region (LRRK2) represent the most common genetic cause of Parkinson's disease. Because LRRK2 is the most common gene defect responsible for Parkinson's disease, it has been a focus of many laboratories. So what does LRRK2 do? One of the jobs of LRRK2 in the brain seems to be to tag proteins. When proteins are tagged, this signals the brain to change its cell manufacturing process. However, when bad LRRK2 tags proteins, it results in over-manufacturing. An excess of proteins can lead to the death of brain cells. Bad LRRK2 performs its tagging function by attaching what have been referred to as phosphate groups. Bad LRRK2 leads to increases in proteins through its action on a part of the cell called ribosomal s15. The Dawson duo demonstrated that removing the phosphate group tagging of s15 prevented degeneration. Further, by administering a low dose of anisomycin, which blocks protein production, the Dawson strategy also rescued flies with LRRK2 mutations.25

Though these findings are exciting, we should remember that they have yet to be translated into humans. The Dawsons suggest that one way to treat LRRK2 Parkinson's disease would be to simply block phosphorylation of the s15 ribosomal protein. This idea may be formulated into a strategy for a future human clinical drug trial. Further, if there is a clinical trial, we will need a way to measure success and to monitor s15 phosphorylation. Phosphorylation could possibly be a blood or other biomarker of bad LRRK2 activity. Additionally, there is interest in a class of drugs called the C-Abl tyrosine kinase inhibitors because of findings in another genetic form of Parkinson's disease called PARKIN. The PARKIN protein is modified by c-Abl and this interaction could be the critical step leading to accumulation of toxic proteins in the brain. C-Abl inhibitors have been proposed as a way to block this protein buildup.26 Though there are many steps remaining in human translation, the findings from these recent works provide something for the Parkinson's community to cheer about.

The following drug therapies have been tried for disease modification or neuroprotection and have not been shown effective for this indication:

- Creatine
- CoQ10
- GLP-1 agonists
- CoganeTM – PYM50028
- Urate
- Sapogenin PYM50028 (steroidal)
- Exendin-4 and liraglutide – GLP agonist
- CX-516 ampakine

*Smokers have been observed in multiple studies to have a lower risk of developing Parkinson's disease, and there has been ongoing interest in nicotine as a disease- modifying approach in Parkinson's disease patients. The α7 nicotinic acetylcholine receptors (nAChRs) may prove useful targets for treatment of dyskinesia and also in slowing disease progression. The nicotine patch is undergoing a large placebo-controlled, randomized, multi-center trial listed on clinicaltrials.gov.

*There is a debate among experts as to whether the 1mg dose of rasagiline is neuroprotective or disease modifying. There was an article in the New England Journal of Medicine recently suggesting this possibility, but this effect was not observed with the 2mg dose.

Blood Tests for Parkinson's Disease

Patients and family members have been waiting for news about the possibility of a blood test to detect Parkinson's disease. A small article was published in the

Federation of American Societies for Experimental Biology Journal. Penelope Foulds and colleagues reported the results of a study that examined phosphory-lated alpha-synuclein as a potential candidate for use as a blood test in the detection of Parkinson's disease.27

Foulds and colleagues focused their investigation on a protein called alpha-synuclein. This protein is thought to be important to the cause of Parkinson's disease and is a critical component in the deposits that accumu-late in the Parkinson's disease brain. The authors measured alpha-synuclein in both Parkinson's disease and in control patients. They reported that Parkinson's disease patients had an abnormal phosphorylated form of alpha-synuclein. The changes in the blood were sampled over a three-month period and were found to be stable in 30 patients.

There were, however, several issues with this study. First, the sample size was too small to conclude that this test will prove viable in a much larger popula-tion of Parkinson's disease patients. Second, the authors provided little informa-tion on the actual patients they studied. Parkinson's disease is not one disease, and as groups develop blood tests, they will need to carefully characterize and re-port the clinical symptoms of the patients studied. Additionally, research groups will need to be cautious in generalizing that all Parkinson's disease patients will reveal blood changes. Finally, changes in phosphorylated alpha-synuclein could possibly occur in other Parkinsonian syndromes, other neurological diseases and other systemic diseases. These other diseases must be carefully investigated. Though there were important methodological issues with this study, it is still likely we will see Parkinson's disease blood tests and biomarkers in the near future.

If successfully developed, how would a blood test for Parkinson's disease be used? There are several potential options for this emerging technology. First, if a disease- modifying therapy can be developed, then identifying at-risk patients for early intervention could be critical. A blood test could potentially identify those at risk and help to facilitate early intervention. Another important use for a blood test could be in monitoring the symptomatic treatment of current Parkinson's disease sufferers, especially in those enrolled in drug trials. The test would, however, need to reflect changes in biological activity over time and would also need to closely correlate to changes in disease state (e.g. progression of symptoms).

A blood test for Parkinson's disease would also introduce important ethical considerations, especially for asymptomatic individuals. Though the test may not reflect genetic status, it may unmask a Parkinson's disease diagnosis. Revealing a potential risk to develop Parkinson's disease could profoundly change a person's life. Studies of genetic counseling have revealed that once patients understand the implications of a blood or a genetic test, they will often decline it. Additionally, for currently symptomatic individuals, close monitoring of disease status could result in stress, anxiety and unnecessary worry that may ultimately translate into a worsened overall quality of life.

It is important to understand that many groups around the world are attempting to develop blood tests and biomarkers for Parkinson's disease. It is likely that many of the methodological limitations of blood tests will soon wane and successful approaches will eventually emerge. As we move forward, it will be important for the field to clearly define the potential uses of a blood test and especially to protect patients and also families. There will likely be more than one blood test in the future, and close communication with an experienced doctor will be critical in deciding which test, or which battery of tests, will be appropriate. In summary, the development of blood tests has the potential to improve the lives of many Parkinson's disease patients and also to push the research horizon in a positive direction. These tests, however, must be pursued cautiously and the important ethical implications considered.[28]

DAT and MRI Scans for Diagnosis and for Tracking Disease Progression

The FDA-approved DaTscan (Ioflupane I 123 injection, also known as phenyltropane) is performed by using a radiopharmaceutical agent that can be injected into a patient's veins in a procedure referred to as SPECT imaging. After injection, the compound can be visualized by a special detector called a gamma camera. The scan measures something called the dopamine active transporter (DAT), and it can help a doctor determine if patients are suffering from Parkinson's disease or from symptoms that look like Parkinson's disease (e.g. parkinsonism). The side effects are minimal (e.g. headache, dizziness, increased appetite and a creepy-crawly feeling under the skin). One of the most frequently asked questions about Parkinson's disease on our worldwide "Ask the Doctor" NPF web-based forum (www.parkinson.org) is whether or not to pursue DAT scanning to confirm a diagnosis of Parkinson's disease.

Currently in most cases of Parkinson's disease, DAT scans are unnecessary for confirmation of the diagnosis, especially if you have seen an expert and you are experiencing a satisfactory response to dopaminergic therapy. In cases where the expert is not sure of the diagnosis, or when potentially risky procedures are being considered (e.g. deep brain stimulation surgery), it is reasonable for your doctor to recommend a DAT scan. It is important to keep in mind that DAT scans should be performed only by experienced centers who have executed a large volume of Parkinson's disease scans because experience is important for accurately interpreting imaging results.

DAT scans examine the "function" of the brain rather than its anatomy. This is an important point because unlike in strokes and tumors, the brain anatomy of a Parkinson's disease patient is largely normal. These scans can show changes in brain chemistry, such as a decrease in dopamine, which can identify Parkinson's disease and other kinds of parkinsonism. PET scans usually focus on glucose (sugar) metabolism, and SPECT/DAT scans focus on the activity of the dopamine transporter. There are several compounds available for use in both PET and SPECT scanning.

The new DAT scans use a substance that "tags" a part of a neuron in the brain where dopamine attaches to it, and it reveals the density of healthy dopamine neurons. Therefore, the more of the picture that "lights up," the more surviving brain cells. Interpretations of DAT can, however, be tricky. The first determination is whether the scan is normal or abnormal. Next, the expert will determine if the scan follows the pattern of Parkinson's disease. Finally, a determination of severity of the brain cell loss will be made.

Recently, it has come to light that in studies where experts attempted to diagnose Parkinson's disease very early in its course (within the first few years of symptoms), a subset of patients have turned up with negative DAT scans. These patients did not develop progressive symptoms of Parkinson's disease. These findings have been humbling, and they lend credence to the importance of following patients carefully over long periods of time to ensure both accurate diagnosis and also appropriate treatment.

DAT should not be routinely used for the diagnosis of Parkinson's disease. Patients with progressive symptoms and an adequate response to Parkinson's disease drugs do not need this expensive imaging. In cases where the diagnosis is uncertain (e.g. Parkinson's disease versus essential tremor), a DAT can be useful. In general, these scans cannot reliably separate Parkinson's disease from parkinsonism (multiple system atrophy, corticobasal degeneration, progressive supranuclear palsy), therefore if you seek a scan, you will still need an expert to sort out your clinical picture and diagnosis.29,30

There are new imaging techniques emerging for Parkinson's disease that may allow us to better quantitate brain-based abnormalities. David Vaillancourt, Ph.D., at the University of Florida has developed a MRI technique that may be able to diagnose and also to track progression of Parkinson's disease. Vaillancourt was interested in whether using MRI to measure free-water content in the substantia nigra could also be used to track disease progression. He studied patients with and without Parkinson's disease. Free-water in the very back portion of the substantia nigra was increased in Parkinson's disease, and he was indeed able to track progression.31 These findings could be useful, not only in diagnosis, but also as a biomarker to measure the effectiveness of neuroprotective drugs in clinical trials.32

Take home points:

- Inosine, Isradipine, and Pioglitzaone are already FDA-approved drugs for other diseases and are promising potential therapies for disease modification and symptomatic treatment of Parkinson's disease. It is possible antimalaria drugs may be repurposed for disease modification and treatment of Parkinson's disease.
- Nilotinab, C-Abl inhibitor drugs, jun-N-terminal kinsases (JNK), antibiotics (e.g. anisomycin) as well as other repurposed medications may have the potential for disease modification in Parkinson's disease.
- Blood tests and imaging studies are being developed to diagnose Parkinson's disease, but there are severe limitations in their effectiveness and universality.
- An imaging biomarker to track disease progression will be important for disease- modifying drug studies.

·⊷═◉ ◉═⊶·

CHAPTER 2

Coffee, Tea, Exercise, Interdisciplinary Teams and Caregivers

I have measured out my life with coffee spoons.

–T.S. Elliot

ONE OF THE exciting recent changes in the treatment approach to Parkinson's disease has been the development of new brain targets that have moved the field beyond the typical dopamine and dopamine agonist-based treatments. One of the brain targets that has gleaned tremendous interest from multiple pharmaceutical companies, as well as from leading scientists from around the world, has been the adenosine A2A receptor. Interestingly, the A2A receptor may underpin the potential benefits of coffee, tea and exercise.

What is the adenosine A2A receptor? There are a group of circuits in the brain called the basal ganglia that are collectively involved in the underlying problems that result in the symptoms of Parkinson's disease. The basal ganglia have a ton of adenosine A2A receptors located on the outside of nerve cells that we refer to as neurons. Many of these receptors have been observed to be co-located next to dopamine receptors. Scientists believe that you can either activate the dopamine receptor, or alternatively, block the adenosine A2 receptor as a way to improve the symptoms of Parkinson's disease. There has been some speculation that this class of drugs may, when used in combination with dopaminergic drugs (e.g. levodopa and agonists), facilitate a reduction in the dosage of dopamine and a coincident reduction in side effects.33,34

Istradefylline is, for example, a pill that is an adenosine A2A receptor antagonist that has been tried in multiple human studies of patients suffering with Parkinson's disease. The results of these studies have revealed a mild beneficial effect on wearing off and on motor fluctuations. Istradefylline did not achieve FDA approval in the United States but has been approved for use in Japan.35-37 Biotie has been investigating another A2A receptor antagonist for Parkinson's disease called tozadenant (SYN115). Early treatment results have revealed improvements in "off" time. Finally, Merck recently investigated another drug called Preladenant. Preladenant is also an adenosine A2A receptor antagonist. Early studies revealed promising effects for this compound on Parkinson's disease related "off" periods. Unfortunately, three separate phase III trials did not provide evidence for efficacy over a placebo pill. Vipadenant (BIIB014) and ST-1535 are two A2A receptor compounds that remain under investigation in animal models for Parkinson's and other diseases. Other compounds known to block the adenosine A2A receptor and have been used in various animal and human studies are: ATL-444, MSX-3, SCH-58261, 412, 348, 442,416, VER-6623, 6947, 7835, ZM-241, 385.

Though drug studies have been disappointing, patients should keep in mind that the A2A receptor may be affected by the intake of caffeine and tea and also by performing exercise. It is exciting that pharmaceutical companies and scientists are beginning to look beyond the dopaminergic system for better therapies to treat those suffering from Parkinson's disease. We should not get too disappointed in the early drug trial failures, as we are just beginning to explore novel and potentially therapeutic areas of the brain that may help this and the next generation of Parkinson's patients. In the meantime, perhaps we should turn our attention to coffee, tea and exercise.38

Adenosine A2A Receptor Drugs in Development

- Istradefylline KW-6002 (Kyowa) – Available in Japan, failed U.S. FDA; may be tried again in future study
- Tozadenant aka SYN115 (Biotie) – Planned upcoming follow-up trial
- Preladenant (Merck) – Phase III trials were disappointing
- Vipadenant (Biogen/Vernalis) – Not currently being pursued
- ST-1535 – This drug has been tried in animals

*Remember to keep in mind that caffeine (coffee) is a widely available adenosine A2A antagonist.

Coffee

Ron Postuma and his colleagues in Canada recently put caffeine to the test as a symptomatic therapy. Postuma designed a simple six-week study that examined daytime sleepiness and effects on motor and non-motor features (tremor, stiffness, slowness as well as depression, anxiety and non-motor features). He focused on patients with the symptom of sleepiness and administered caffeine pills at either 100 mg twice daily or 200 mg twice daily. He carefully controlled the experiment by administering a caffeine placebo pill to a group of patients. Interestingly, caffeine did not help sleepiness, but it did improve the motor symptoms of Parkinson's disease. There was some suggestion that at low doses caffeine was more effective against motor symptoms when compared to the higher doses.[39,40] There has also been a suggestion that the positive effects of coffee are more pronounced in men than women. So the great news for Parkinson's disease patients is that coffee in moderation may be helpful as a symptomatic therapy.

Tea

Tea is an ancient, centuries-old beverage that is consumed by virtually all of the world's population. Tea is composed of polyphenols, methylxanthine, caffeine, fats, amino acids and other substances. Tea has been thought to reduce cancer risk, prevent heart disease and even aid in weight loss. The flavonoids, caffeine and theanine have been tested in animal models of Parkinson's disease and have shown protection against cell loss in similar areas of the brain that are affected in the human Parkinson's patient. A recent meta analysis of all studies on tea and Parkinson's risk has revealed that across 1,418 cases and 4,250 control patients, there was a protective effect of tea drinking on Parkinson's disease risk. Interestingly, whether you drink one or more cups a day did not impact the risk.[41,42]

Louis Tan, one of the authors of the Singapore Chinese Health study, reported differential effects of black versus green tea. People in his study who drank at most one cup of black tea a day (but not green tea) decreased their risk of developing Parkinson's disease. Caffeine also reduced the risk of Parkinson's disease. This study lends support to the mounting evidence supporting a caffeine Parkinson's-related benefit. Interestingly, most black teas have more caffeine than green teas.[43]

What should patients understand about coffee and tea drinking and Parkinson's disease? Consumption of coffee or tea seems to reduce the risk of developing Parkinson's disease. Once you have been diagnosed with Parkinson's disease, no matter how much time you spend in Starbucks, you can no longer alter your risk profile. The cat is out of the bag. Consumption of caffeine in moderate doses does however seem to benefit the motor symptoms of Parkinson's disease.

Exercise

The recent surge in publications on Parkinson's disease-related exercise has left many patients and doctors ill equipped to implement practical programs. Most of the exercise trials in Parkinson's disease have revealed meaningful benefits both in Parkinson's specific symptoms and in quality of life. Though we have yet to sort out the best types of exercise regimes, the most appropriate frequency of exercise and the optimal intensity of therapy for any individual patient, there is unfortunately an even larger issue facing the field. Many people suffering from Parkinson's disease do not exercise. Understanding the barriers preventing implementation of a regular Parkinson's disease exercise program will be important for both prescribing clinicians and patients.

Terry Ellis and colleagues in the journal Physical Therapy explored the barriers to exercise in community-dwelling people with Parkinson's disease. The authors studied 260 Parkinson's disease patients and compared exercisers to non-exercisers. The patients were asked to complete the barriers subscale of the Physical Fitness and Exercise Activity Levels of Older Adults Scale. The study revealed that in people who did not exercise, there was a low expectation for positive benefit. The non-exercise group also was concerned about the amount of time needed per day to initiate such a program as well as the fall risk.44

Making our clinicians and our patients aware of the barriers to implementing exercise programs for Parkinson's disease will aid us in overcoming the issues unearthed by Terry Ellis. There will, in the near future, likely be more Parkinson's-specific research studies that will shed even more light on this issue. Education will play a pivotal role in facilitating the implementation of exercise plans, and health care practitioners as well as family members should be prepared to present Parkinson's disease patients with recent scientific data. A higher level conversation about exercise, citing its proven benefits, has an enhanced potential to reverse some of the low expectations expressed by many Parkinson's patients. Additionally, it should be stressed to patients that consistent daily exercise may be performed in small portions of time (30 to 60 minutes a day) and in many cases in the home setting. Finally, there are many exercises that can be performed safely without increasing the fall risk. Involvement of a physical therapist and a care partner can be useful in setting up a safe and consistent home-based or gym-based program.

As more studies clarify the types of exercise we should be prescribing for individual patients, more clinicians will need to develop strategies to defeat the barriers to implementing exercise programs. Exercise is likely to improve the quality of life for most Parkinson's disease patients, but we must meet the public health challenge to achieve adoption and implementation by the Parkinson's disease community.

Lisa Shulman and colleagues at the University of Maryland compared treadmill exercises, stretching and resistance exercises as a treatment for walking, strength and fitness in Parkinson's disease. There were 67 patients tested, and the lower-intensity settings for treadmill walking were better than stretching, resistance exercises and even a higher-intensity treadmill training. Predictably only the use of stretching and resistance training have improved measures of strength. Shulman and colleagues concluded a low- intensity workout on the treadmill paired with resistance exercises had the potential to be the most beneficial combination for Parkinson's disease patients.45

Meanwhile, Dan Corcos at the Northwestern University National Parkinson Foundation Center of Excellence in Chicago took a different approach than Shulman and colleagues. Corcos was interested in a set of weight lifting tasks referred to as progressive resistance exercises, and he wanted to compare this approach to standard stretching, balance and strengthening routines in Parkinson's disease patients. The progressive resistance exercises showed more benefit than traditional stretching, balance and strengthening exercises.46

Jay Alberts at the Cleveland Clinic took yet another approach to exercise in Parkinson's disease. Alberts was interested in the animal studies showing that forced exercise improved motor function. He also put this to the test many years ago when he pedaled a tandem bike across Iowa with a Parkinson's disease patient in the rear seat. He hypothesized that the forced exercise was the reason for her dramatic improvements during the charity ride. He then performed a small, controlled experiment in which patients pedaled at a rate 30 percent greater than their typical rate. He compared the outcomes to a different group of Parkinson's patients pedaling at their typical rate. Although the aerobic fitness improved for both sets of patients, the forced exercise group improved their Parkinson's motor scores by 35 percent, and the typical rate pedal group did not improve.47

Though this approach has been adopted by many Parkinson's patients, and the initial Alberts patient was actually one I followed at Emory, we have advocated caution in taking this approach. Several of our patients have pushed themselves too hard and actually worsened their Parkinson's symptoms. It is important that your doctor and your physical therapist help choose the appropriate exercise, the right dose (frequency) and the safest approach for your exercise regimen.48

The Parkinson's Care Team

One of the most common questions we hear from patients is: "What can I do to be sure I am getting the best possible treatment for my Parkinson's disease?" Most doctors focus on treatment-based recommendations (e.g. drugs, exercise, diet, etc.). The initial answer to "the best" treatment question may start with "making sure you are co-managed by both a neurologist and a primary care physician."

Allison Willis and colleagues at the University of Pennsylvania National Parkinson Foundation Center of Excellence asked the provocative question of whether involving a neurologist in the care of a Parkinson's disease patient made a difference in outcome. In a careful review of 138,000 Parkinson's disease Medicare beneficiaries followed between 2002-2005, they discovered that only 68 percent of Parkinson's disease patients received neurologist care, with the remainder receiving only primary care. Willis observed that neurologist-treated patients were "less likely to be placed in a skilled nursing facility, had a lower risk of hip fracture, and had a lower adjusted likelihood of death." Another interesting finding was that women and minorities received less specialty care. The diagnosis of Parkinson's disease was not confirmed by a specialist in this study, and data was not available to ascertain whether patients actually saw a Parkinson's disease specialist.49,50

In an age when patients and clinicians seek more expensive diagnostic tests, it is intriguing to consider that a simple referral to a neurologist for co-management with a primary care physician may have the biggest and most important impact on a Parkinson's disease patient's outcome. In a way, this finding should not be surprising. After all, the best diagnostic test for Parkinson's disease remains an expert neurological examination, and it would therefore logically follow that the best chance for clinical optimization of the patient would be with a neurologist. A Parkinson's disease patient is complex, and motor, non-motor, behavioral, and in some cases surgical options must be considered for the best overall management. The pharmacological strategies for Parkinson's disease are complicated and often require multiple medications, multiple doses and medication intervals as close as every two to three hours. Despite the limitations in the methodology of this type of study (drawing data from Medicare beneficiaries), if the findings are true and confirmed, there could be a tremendous economic savings to the health care system by simply executing a referral and co-managing with a general neurologist. Perhaps an even better recommendation would be for co-management by a Parkinson's disease neurologist; however, Medicare does not provide funds for training Parkinson's disease specialists as they do for cardiologists and other medical specialties. Consequently, there is a critical shortage of Parkinson's disease-trained specialists.51

Despite this shortage in specialists, I always remember what Maya Angelou said: "I've learned that people will forget what you said, people will forget what you did, but people will never forget how you made them feel."6 At our center, we have trained over 40 Parkinson's doctors, and we constantly remind them that every member of the team, including the schedulers, check-in staff and nurses, must all embrace the vision of a truly patient-centric Parkinson's care experience.

Caregiver Strain

It is widely appreciated that one of the keys to success for many patients with Parkinson's disease is a fully-engaged caregiver. Caregivers play an important role, due to the impact of the disease but also to the complexity of home care regimens. Caregiving is not easy, it's not sexy and it can be a full time, 24/7 job. It can be difficult for a spouse who is also a caregiver to watch the transformation of a loved one. Helen Keller's caregiver Anne Sullivan was once quoted as saying;

"I cannot explain it; but when difficulties arise, I am not perplexed or doubtful. I know how to meet them." We have been striving at the National Parkinson Foundation to help the community better identify and more effectively meet the challenges of caregiver strain. In our current Parkinson's Outcomes Project Quality Improvement Initiative (QII) study, we have assembled the largest longitudinal cohort of Parkinson's disease patients ever followed in the setting of a clinical study. We have been collecting a measure called the multi-dimensional caregiver strain index on all of the spouses and caregivers, and we have learned that recognizing and treating caregiver strain is critical.

Tanya Simuni at the NPF Center of Excellence at Northwestern University examined the impact that caregiver strain had on patients in our large Parkinson's Outcome Study. The single most important factor impacting strain was quality of life, and in particular, mobility-related quality of life. High caregiver strain was associated with later stage disease, presence of concomitant medications (such as antidepressants and antipsychotics), social work visits, male gender and decreased cognition. Overall, there was a high prevalence of caregiver strain, and the impact on quality of life was huge.52

We also recently sought to identify the potential impact of the change in a regular caregiver on health-related quality of life (HRQL). We reasoned that a change in caregiver may impact both health and well-being. We examined baseline and one year follow-up data on 3,454 subjects. A change in a caregiver was reported in 104 subjects (5.3 percent), with 50 changing to no caregiver, 26 to another family member, 26 to a paid caregiver and 2 to another caregiver. Overall, those whose caregiver status changed reported a diminished quality of life, and some even had worsening on a motor walking task. This study taught us that when the caregiver situation changes, it is important to consider the impact on quality of life.

Finally, Julie Carter at our NPF Center of Excellence at Oregon Health & Science University studied the impact of motor and non-motor Parkinson's disease symptoms on caregiver strain and depression. In a sample of 219 spouse caregivers, her research team demonstrated that Parkinson's patient's symptoms were important predictors of caregiver strain and depression. Interestingly, the non-motor psychological symptoms had a greater impact on caregiver strain.[53,54]

The take home message for our patients, families and medical teams attempting to manage Parkinson's disease is to be aware that caregiver strain is extremely common. It is important to identify and address not only the motor and non-motor symptoms of Parkinson's disease but also caregiver strain. Treatment has a high likelihood of improving quality of life. Remember at each visit to the doctor, many times the health and well-being of the caregiver should be considered just as important as the health and well-being of the Parkinson's disease patient.

Take Home Points:

- Coffee, tea and exercise can be potentially beneficial in Parkinson's disease risk and symptomatic treatment.
- The mechanisms of action for coffee, tea and exercise are likely non-dopaminergic and at least partially mediated by the brain's adenosine receptors.
- There are barriers to exercise, and education is important to helping overcome these barriers.
- Referral to a neurologist, and if available, a specialty neurologist can improve outcomes.
- A team-based approach (neurologist, psychiatrist, social worker, health counselor, counseling psychologist) to care that involves identification and treatment of caregiver strain can improve outcomes.

⋯⊨◉ ◉⊨⋯

CHAPTER 3

Extended Release/Novel Delivery Systems for Parkinson's Disease Drug and When to Start Drug Therapy

"Techno-optimism is a belief in the power of technology to extend our sphere of possibilities and, ultimately, a belief that technology helps us solve and transcend problems, limitations and obstacles."

–Jason Silva

ONE OF THE most exciting aspects of medicine and of medical research has been the direct translation of discoveries from bench to bedside. In the 1950s, Arvid Carlsson rescued animals with parkinsonian symptoms by utilizing a new chemical compound called L-Dopa. Carlsson's work led to his Nobel Prize in 2000. In the late 1960s, his observations were translated into humans by George Cotzias, and the drug L-Dopa instantly became one of the most remarkable treatments ever introduced for a human neurological disease. In 1988, the combination drug known as Sinemet (carbidopa/levodopa) was approved by the FDA, and millions of Parkinson's disease patients have enormously benefited.55

In the early years, the knowledge in the best use of Sinemet had not been fully realized or even understood. Paralleling the discovery and use of this drug was the blossoming subspecialty of neurology, now referred to as movement disorders. Movement disorders-trained neurologists embraced Sinemet and used it to refine the treatment of Parkinson's disease patients. They became skilled at tailoring therapy to improve individual and highly-specific symptoms. As a specialty, they made important observations and published many seminal papers. Amazingly, thousands of patients with this previously devastating neurodegenerative condition began surviving 20 plus years, thus even general doctors began commonly prescribing Sinemet.

As patients with Parkinson's disease survived longer and longer on new Sinemet drug regimens, scientists and physicians began to better understand the titration of dosages, and the efficient management of patients. It was obvious to the medical field that in expert hands, adjustment of medication dosages and medication intervals was intimately tied to the short and long term success for individual Parkinson's disease patients. It also was clear that the drug Sinemet was safe and tolerable in nearly every case.

One of the most frustrating aspects of care for the Parkinson's disease patient is the constant re-dosing of dopaminergic medications. Parkinson's is unlike any other disease. As brain cells are gradually lost over the course of many years, the frequency of dosages and sometimes the doses themselves must be adjusted to assure adequate improvement of symptoms. These adjustments can be complex, and often they require frequent trips to an experienced neurologist. One important area of research has been the investment into technologies aimed at extending the life of dopaminergic therapies thereby reducing the need for frequent re-dosing.

In the late 1980s and early 1990s clinicians and researchers converged on an idea to extend the life of the common drug called Sinemet. In Latin, Sinemet translates into "sin" which means without and "emet" which means vomit. Sinemet has two components: carbidopa and levodopa. The carbidopa blocks an enzyme called dopamine decarboxylase which when administered with levodopa controls nausea and facilitates more dopamine delivery to the brain. Ipecac, which was given for many years in emergency rooms to address drug overdoses by stimulating vomiting, is essentially a form of dopamine. Once the tolerability issue had been addressed, extending the half-life of the drug became the next critical and most logical step. Efforts in this direction have been underway for three decades.

Peter LeWitt from the Henry Ford Hospital in Detroit discussed the current state of the field in 1992. LeWitt pointed out that Sinemet was absorbed in the small intestine and metabolized over a period of approximately three to four hours. Sinemet CR, which was a sustained-release preparation, was purported to double the effect. In one early trial of 25 patients fewer daily dosages of medication were required. Unfortunately, these early studies did not recognize the complexity of predicting half-lives of drugs in a disease in which brain cells and brain circuitry is in a dynamic state of change.56,57

Today most experts recognize that the CR formulations have not lived up to the hype. Many patients have reported no differences when switching between formulations, especially if they have had disease for five or more years. One distinct advantage for CR formulations has been observed in a subset of patients with what has been called peak-dose dyskinesia. Dyskinetic movements are bothersome, extra dance-like movements that occur when the medication is absorbed and reaches its highest level in the bloodstream. CR preparations have lower peaks than regular release formulations, and these lower peaks may be better for avoiding the dyskinetic movements.

Most practitioners use one formulation or the other (regular vs. CR), and now more than 20 years after its introduction into the field, Sinemet CR can be judged as falling short of a major advance. One of my former fellows, Amanda Thompson Avila, who joined us from Brown University joked that her patients tell her the CR stands for crappy.

One interesting and useful formulation of Sinemet that was approved in 2004 is Parcopa. Parcopa is essentially Sinemet, but it is manufactured as a dissolvable tablet, therefore can be useful for some patients who have trouble swallowing pills or taking medications by mouth. Parcopa essentially works in the same way as Sinemet, and the half-life of the drug and absorption properties are nearly identical.58

In 2015, we frequently hear from Parkinson's disease patients that current carbidopa/levodopa medication preparations fail to adequately address disease-related symptoms. The cited medication shortcomings include: 1) medication dosages taking too long to "kick in" and start working, 2) medication wearing off before the next scheduled dose, 3) severe on-off medication fluctuation periods (e.g. rapid cycling during the day ranging from feeling completely on medication to completely off medication), 4) dyskinesia (too much movement, usually resulting from too high of a blood level of dopamine), 5) too many pills and 6) too many medication dosage intervals (e.g. taking medications every one to two hours throughout the waking day). Patients also have other issues that levodopa does not address including walking, balance, talking and thinking issues, but these will likely require a totally different approach rather than simple levodopa replacement.

Robert Hauser at the National Parkinson Foundation Center of Excellence at the University of South Florida, along with colleagues from 68 North American and European study sites, recently published a paper on a new extended release formulation of carbidopa/levodopa (IPX066, now named Rytary).59,60 The new formulation is different from its predecessors. It contains special beads designed to dissolve at different rates within the stomach and the intestines. The medication capsule was designed to provide a longer lasting benefit for patients with Parkinson's disease. This current randomized study included 393 Parkinson's disease patients who reported at least two and a half hours of "off time," defined as periods when they felt the medication was not working. The authors aimed to improve the number of hours of "off time" each day for patients randomized to the new extended release formulation as compared to the older and standard regular release carbidopa/levodopa. The results revealed that the group on the extended release formulation took fewer overall medication dosages (3.6 vs. 5 doses per day), however, they also took more total pills. The daily "off time" improved by over an hour each day in the extended release formulation. Both medications in this trial were safe and well tolerated.60

If we return to the six areas in which Parkinson's disease patients have been seeking improved medication formulations, Rytary was observed to improve issues in two categories: wearing off between dosages and improvement by increasing the time interval between dosages. The results of the current study cannot be widely applied to patients with severe dyskinesia, severe on-off fluctuations or later stage disease. The new extended release formulation was also observed to increase the total bloodstream levodopa exposure by 30 to 40 percent as compared to conventional immediate release levodopa. Increasing levodopa in the bloodstream is thought to decrease the threshold for dyskinesia, as has been observed with other Parkinson's drugs such as Entacapone and Stalevo. Although dosed less frequently, the extended release formulation actually required more total pills per day. The authors felt that a newer formulation of the same drug, which they anticipate will be used in clinical practice, could in the future facilitate a decrease in pill number.

Patients and families should be excited by the news that a new formulation of carbidopa/levodopa is now FDA approved and available. However, patients and clinicians should also be aware that there are limitations and caution should be exercised, especially since the new formulation could lower the dyskinesia threshold. Our experience has been that Rytary works best when trying to maintain a patient on three times a day dosing rather than adding a fourth dose. It may be challenging to titrate Rytary in more complex situations. Dosages and dosage intervals of any formulation of carbidopa/levodopa, including Rytary, should be carefully adjusted at each clinic visit to address changes in Parkinson's symptoms. The success or failure of dopamine replacement therapy is more dependent on the expert adjusting the therapy than the formulation. It is good news that drug manufacturers are now listening to Parkinson's disease patients and trying to address their six major concerns, although it would seem obvious there is a lot of room for improvement.61

The novel forms of levodopa (dopamine) in development are:

- Rytary IPX0666 (recently FDA approved)
- Duopa Continuous infusion gel (recently FDA approved)
- Accordion Pill (IntecPharma) – Layered polymer sheaths for better GI absorption
- XP21279 (XenoPort) – Nutritional receptors to improve absorption
- NDO612, L-dopa Pump patch (NeuroDerm) – Pump patch to improve delivery
- SD-1077, Deuterated L-dopa (Auspex) – Prolongs duration of action in the brain
- CVT-301 Inhaled L-dopa (Civitas) – Inhaled dopamine dry powder
- Levodopa Methyl ester, Melevodopa – Not currently being pursued

Generic Medications

It is important for the Parkinson's disease patient to be "aware in care." Inactive drug ingredients, and especially color dyes often employed in pill manufacturing, can cause adverse events. Serious hypersensitivity reactions have been reported from use of such common dyes. An unfortunate medication-related circumstance was recently reported to the National Parkinson Foundation Ask the Doctor service. A patient reported that shortly after switching from a blue Sinemet CR 25/100 to a yellow generic formulation, he experienced swelling of the face, lips and mouth. Similarly, we are aware of other patients who have reported rashes when making similar switches. It turns out that the yellow dye commonly present in the generic form of Sinemet (carbidopa/levodopa) can possibly but rarely be responsible for these types of side effects. If you suspect a pill color allergy, you should contact your doctor, and be aware that yellow dye allergies may occur more commonly in patients who are also allergic to aspirin. The treatment for the allergy is simply to contact your doctor and make a change to a blue pill formulation. Some sensitive patients will benefit from avoidance of yellow dyes in the diet.62

In 2010 and 2011 there was a national shortage of Sinemet. This occurred as the brand for carbidopa/levodopa was transitioned from Merck to Mylan. The transition resulted in a worrisome and short-lived drug shortage. When generic formulations became available, multiple complaints were reported to the National Parkinson Foundation Helpline. These complaints ranged from weaker efficacy of the generic drug, worsening of motor fluctuations, dyskinesia, allergy and skin rash. We reminded patients that when switching to a generic formulation, there may be as much as a 20 percent difference in treatment effect. Sometimes, however, a generic may be desired, especially in Parkinson's disease patients who experience dyskinesia from tiny medication dosages. (Some people have referred to these cases as "brittle" Parkinson's disease dyskinesia.) One should remember that FDA approval of a brand name drug requires demonstration of its pharmacokinetics, efficacy, safety and tolerability in both a healthy population and also in the Parkinson's disease population. In contrast, approval of a generic drug only requires demonstrating its bioequivalence in the blood but not the demonstration of a clinical treatment effect in Parkinson's disease.[62]

Another important Sinemet issue has been the myth that there is a maximum dose that must never be exceeded. It may be a shock to learn that the 1988 FDA recommendation not to exceed eight tablets of Sinemet a day has never been revised.[63,64] The original document is so antiquated that most Parkinson's disease patients and families will find the information contained within it somewhat laughable. The document recommends taking one Sinemet tablet three times a day initially and ultimately recommends not to exceed two tablets four times a day. The document also states that "a significant proportion of infant rats of both sexes are expected to die at a dose of 800 mg/kg." Modern Parkinson's disease patients and their physicians understand that the management of the individual patient must be carefully tailored. The brain's dopamine supply in Parkinson's disease is slowly depleted, and to correct the deficiency, multiple doses of Sinemet sometimes administered as frequently as one and two hours apart may be necessary to restore quality of life and to facilitate the basic reintegration back into society.

Unfortunately, patients and families are not laughing at the 1988 FDA recommendations, as Medicare and insurance providers have been denying prescriptions for Sinemet and for generic carbidopa/levodopa when they exceed eight tablets a day.63,64 I think it is safe to say that it is time for the FDA to revise its eight Sinemet a day rule and allow patients and families to realize the full benefits of Arvid Carlsson's remarkable discovery. We recently publicly called for the FDA to revise the eight Sinemet a day rule. The advent of electronic medical records has been compounding this difficult issue for patients, as automatic limits are now being set by nationalized computer systems. Once limits are in computer systems, they can be challenging for individual patients to change. If your insurance carrier or pharmacy blocks filling of your Sinemet prescription purely based on number of daily pills, we suggest you contact your doctor, send an appeal letter and also contact the National Parkinson Foundation Patient Assistance Helpline (1-800-4PD-INFO).65

Dopamine Agonists and a Potential Advantage for the Patch

The early 1980s brought to fruition and to market a new class of drugs. These were the "super" dopamine drugs. Sinemet was a simple replacement therapy, but these super drugs known as dopamine agonists had longer half-lives and directly tickled the brain's dopamine receptors (agonists tickle the brain's receptors and dopamine antagonists like Haldol block them). Pergolide was the first such drug (agonist) to achieve FDA approval.

The mechanism of action for dopamine agonists is the direct stimulation of the brain's dopamine receptors. The mechanism of action of a dopamine agonist is different from levodopa, which is simply a neurotransmitter (i.e. dopamine chemical) replacement strategy. Dopamine agonists, along with levodopa, are the most commonly-utilized drugs to address the motor symptoms of Parkinson's disease. Dopamine agonists became popular over the last decade after it was suggested that there may be benefits to their use in early disease. The past several years, however, have led to a marked reduction in the popularity and use of dopamine agonists by Parkinson's disease experts. The reduction in use has been mainly driven by the recognition of the many troublesome side effects including most commonly sleepiness, edema (i.e. swelling), orthostasis (i.e. dizziness), cognitive issues, hallucinations and also the emergence of impulse control disorders (e.g. gambling, shopping, eating, hypersexuality). It is important to keep in mind that dopamine agonists remain an important part of the armamentarium used to treat Parkinson's disease, even if they are not appropriate for all patients. Their use should be carefully monitored by an experienced neurologist.6,66-69

Several pharmaceutical companies over the years have entered the market with different dopamine agonist products. Interestingly, Pergolide was removed from the market in 2007 when it was discovered that the ergot component in the drug was contributing to scarring of the cardiac valves in humans.70 The industry would be dominated by Ropinirole, which was backed by a large study published in the New England Journal of Medicine and Pramipexole, which was similarly backed by a study in JAMA. Though the side effect profile was worse than Sinemet, these drugs had longer half-lives and some studies pointed to the possibility that long-term complications of levodopa could be postponed.71,72 Unfortunately, though patients were highly satisfied on dopamine agonists, it took several years for us to understand that one in six patients could develop an impulse control disorder on this class of drugs.73

Impulse control disorders including behaviors such as gambling, shopping, pathological eating and hypersexuality can occur in one out of every six Parkinson's disease patients taking a dopamine agonist drug. Since these drugs can in many cases be critical for optimization of care in Parkinson's disease, it is important that we develop strategies for their safe use and for appropriate monitoring.

Pedro Garcia-Ruiz and colleagues conducted a study using 2.7 million serious domestic and foreign adverse drug events reported to the FDA between 2003 and 2012. There were 710 events reported for dopamine receptor agonist drugs and 870 for other dopamine receptor drugs. The agonist drugs were strongly associated with impulse control disorders. Two of the most common drugs used in Parkinson's disease, Pramipexole and Ropinerole, had the strongest associations.74

It was clear that the dopamine agonists were strongly associated with the occurrence of impulse control disorders. We decided to ask Peter Schmidt, Ph.D., who runs NPF's Parkinson's Outcomes Project (QII), if he had collected any data from NPF centers that could ultimately inform better Parkinson care.75 Schmidt determined the outcomes for Parkinson's disease patients in his study by using a composite of six important research measures he collected across NPF centers: PDQ-39 (quality of life), TUG (walking), cognition (thinking), caregiver strain, falls and hospitalization. Schmidt's results informed us that more judicious use of dopamine agonists across the NPF Centers of Excellence was associated with better outcomes but only to a certain point. Interesting was the finding that the best centers (i.e. those who achieved the most optimal outcomes), were actually heavy users of dopamine agonists. Schmidt taught us that some of the worst outcomes were seen in the centers using the agonists the least, so experience may have also been an important factor.

It is now without doubt that dopamine agonists are associated with impulse control disorders. Data from the FDA and many other sources support this association. One important piece of information missing from recent studies is the notion that the dopamine agonist patch, Rotigotine, may have a lower incidence of impulse control issues. This is something that we should all keep in mind. Two large, recent studies have shown this diminished incidence, and though it is unclear why, it may have something to do with the continuous delivery system.76 Pramipexole and Ropinerole have both answered with their own extended release formulations, but large-scale direct comparisons have not been performed.

Both clinical experience and the NPF study support the idea that dopamine agonist use can be a powerful adjunct to the best Parkinson's therapy, but clinicians prescribing dopamine agonists should inform patients and caregivers and should proactively monitor for behavioral disorders, just as I do in my clinic. Remember also that the patients suffering from impulse control issues may not have insight into the behavioral problems, and this lack of insight underscores the importance of involving caregivers in any proactive monitoring plan.

Finally, this is an example of the art versus the science of care. Based on the FDA analysis alone, if we had to make a rule about the use of dopamine agonists, that rule would be to use them sparingly. The NPF data, however, tells us that in the hands of a true expert, appropriate use of dopamine agonists can potentially shift patients from good care to great care. Dr. Schmidt and I have been working together to help people with Parkinson's disease to understand the importance of expert care, and the dopamine agonist situation illustrates the importance and complexity of these issues. The best results don't come from simple rules; they come from an informed and tailored approach based on solid data drawn from our community of Parkinson's disease patients.

One other form of rapidly-acting dopamine agonist is apomorphine. Apomorphine has been available for many years and is especially useful for un-predictable "off" medication timing. One disadvantage of this therapy has been the need for subcutaneous injections. A new formulation, APL-130277, a sub-lingual or under-the-tongue version, is currently in clinical trials.77-81

COMT Inhibitors

Another question that has been recently asked is whether we can extend the life of Sinemet by pairing it with another drug. Scientists answered with a pill called a Catechol O-methyltransferase inhibitor. The first of these drugs called Tolcapone was very powerful and useful in improving the action of Sinemet and reducing motor fluctuations. However, in 1998 a handful of patients experi-enced liver failure, and the FDA removed Tolcapone from the market. Though the drug returned to the market with special monitoring precautions, it fell out of general use, even among experts. Entacapone was a safer alternative, and many practitioners turned to this formulation. In 2003, it became available as a single pill with a combination of Sinemet and Entacapone (Stalevo). There was a decade-long speculation that using a COMT inhibitor, thereby promoting continuous drug delivery, would decrease motor fluctuations and dykinesia.82 The STRIDE-PD study in 2010, however, revealed a worse outcome for the more than 300 patients randomized to Stalevo. Therefore, most experts now reduce the amount of Sinemet when considering Stalevo as an approach to extend the life of Sinemet.83 A new COMT inhibitor, Opicapone, is currently being tested in a clinical trials setting. Preliminary data has revealed the possibility that Opicapone may have a more prolonged effect on COMT, extend the bioavailability of Sinemet and may potentially be a safer and more effective alternative to currently available COMT drugs.84

MAO-B Inhibitors

This class of drugs has been used for many years for the symptomatic treatment of Parkinson's disease and also for the potential neuroprotective effects, though the latter remains to be substantiated. There was a recent paper in the New England Journal of Medicine suggesting that use of the 1 mg dose of Rasagiline once daily had potential disease-modifying or neuroprotective effects.85,86 We frequently prescribe these drugs particularly early in the course of Parkinson's disease. When there is an issue of affordability we may switch to the twice a day formulation of a generic MAO-B called Selegiline, which is available as a pill, or more recently in a more expensive dissolvable tablet (Zydis Selegiline). Selegiline has an amphetamine metabolite, and some practitioners believe this is an advantage (alertness, mood, energy), but others have argued that there is no selective advantage. One large early study of Selegiline by the Parkinson Study Group called DATATOP did suggest a better long term outcome in gait for those on this therapy.87

A new MAO-B inhibitor Safinamide is still in clinical trials. Safinamide has a very tight affinity for the MAO-B receptor and not the MAO-A receptor. Stimulation of the MAO-A receptor can lead to side effects. Safinamide also blocks dopamine reuptake as well as sodium and potassium channels and stops a chemical called glutamate from being released. In addition to mild symptomatic effects, there is some interest as to whether Safinomide lasts in the bloodstream for a very long time, thus possibly being helpful for fatigue, mood and thinking issues in Parkinson's disease. There are ongoing studies aimed to demonstrate some of these benefits with Safinomide, but to date it has not been shown to be better than Rasagline or Selegiline.88

Regardless of the MAO-B inhibitor you may choose there is final point that has led to much stress for patients, pharmacists and caregivers. The combination of low dose MAO-B drugs (Rasagiline 1mg or Selegiline 10mg daily) and antidepressants (SSRI's and SNRI's) and the fear of an adverse event may lead pharmacists to refuse to fill prescriptions. The weight of the evidence and as well as tens of thousands of patient experiences has collectively shown that combining low dose MAO-B inhibitors in Parkinson's disease is safe when mixing with antidepressants. If your pharmacist is in doubt show him or her this chapter, and remind them that the big issue is with mixing MAO-A inhibitors with antidepressants (and not MAO-B's).

When Should I Start a Medication for Parkinson's Disease?

Since there is not a proven neuroprotective therapy for Parkinson's disease, when should you start medications? The most important factor in initiating Parkinson's disease medications for an individual patient is whether Parkinson's symptoms affect quality of life, or alternatively, whether symptoms affect work performance. Bothersome Parkinson's symptoms commonly include motor issues (tremor, stiffness, slowness, walking and balance problems) and non-motor issues (depression, anxiety, sexual dysfunction and other issues). Most experts agree that there is no benefit to delaying medication therapy if bothersome symptoms appear. There are also risks in delaying treatment, especially if a treatment delay results in unsteadiness, falls and fractures.

Over the last 10 to 20 years the thinking has evolved regarding when and how to initiate medication therapy for early Parkinson's disease. Most experts agree that the medication dosage and timing of the medication dosage should be carefully monitored in order to maximize the control of responsive

Parkinson-related symptoms. The recommendation that patients should be started on dopamine agonists instead of levodopa (Sinemet, Madopar, Parcopa, Rytary) has faded over the last decade, especially with the emergence of side effects such as leg swelling, nausea and impulse control disorders.

The best advice we can offer Parkinson's disease patients is to not fear treatment or dopaminergic therapy. Sinemet and other Parkinson's therapies have not been shown to be toxic or to accelerate disease progression.89 Dopaminergics never "stop working;" however, they may require adjustment in dose and frequency of administration over time. If Parkinson's disease symptoms affect quality of life or work performance, or if there is a risk of falling, treatment should be initiated. Many practitioners will start with a Monoamine Oxidase B (MAO-B) drug (selegiline, rasagiline, dissolvable selegiline, other), but Parkinson's patients should be aware that the symptomatic effects of MAO-Bs are extremely mild. It is rare to remain on this type of drug without other dopaminergic drugs for any significant period of time. Dopamine agonists (ropinirole, pramipexole, cabergoline, rotigotine, others) and levodopa (Sinemet, Madopar, Parcopa, Rytary) are both excellent choices for early Parkinson's disease therapy. The choice of agent should be weighed only after consideration of the comprehensive medical picture (age, co-morbidities, types of symptoms, history of neurological/psychiatric issues). Therapy should not be viewed as "one size fits all." Finally, patients should remember that if depression, anxiety and other issues persist following dopaminergic treatment, antidepressant therapy may also be warranted.

Other drugs, like amantadine, may also be used in early Parkinson's disease therapy; however, most practitioners reserve amantadine for treatment of dyskinesia, which usually occurs later in the disease course. Patients should keep in mind that exercise is like a drug and that a daily routine is often a great symptomatic supplement to any medication regimen. Many practitioners defer utilization of physical therapy, occupational therapy and speech therapy to later years in the disease; however, these modalities can be powerful treatments when employed early. Finally, all Parkinson's disease patients should have a general practitioner and a dermatologist involved with their care. The reason for involving "other doctors" is because with adequate Parkinson's treatment, a patient will be more likely to encounter difficulties with other medical illnesses (heart disease, prostate cancer, breast cancer, melanoma, etc.). Melanoma, for example, occurs more frequently in Parkinson's disease patients. The increased risk of melanoma is not related to dopaminergic therapy.90,91

Levodopa (Dopamine) Phobia

Many Parkinson's disease patients and family members have been unnecessarily alarmed by the persistent and continuing reports that Sinemet and/or Madopar (the European version of Sinemet) may accelerate disease progression. There have been myths that increasing doses and decreasing the times between drug intervals will lead to toxicity. These reports have been fueled by sparse human evidence. Patients and families should be aware that dopamine replacement therapies such as Sinemet and Madopar are the single most effective and single most important treatments for Parkinson's disease worldwide.

The journal Neurology published an article in 2011 citing important evidence that dopamine replacement therapy was not toxic and did not accelerate disease progression. Laura Parkkinen and colleagues at the National Hospital for Neurology and Neurosurgery, Queen Square in London examined pathology in 96 Parkinson's disease brains donated for research purposes after death. These investigators paired the brain tissue with clinical information including the amount of levodopa used. The study concluded that in the human condition "chronic use of L-dopa does not enhance progression of Parkinson's pathology."

In an accompanying editorial, two prominent neurologists in the field pointed out that there "remains lingering concerns as to whether levodopa is toxic to dopamine neurons and accelerates the degenerative process." The science quoted to support these claims has included levodopa undergoing auto-oxidation and forming reactive oxygen species and toxic protofibrils.92 Additionally, the science includes a classical experiment that showed toxicity when levodopa was mixed with brain cells placed in a dish. The research, however, has fallen short in demonstrating any toxicity of dopamine in the human form of Parkinson's disease. There now exists broad evidence from many studies across many countries (including most recently the ELLDOPA study) that levodopa is beneficial to the human patient and that levodopa has a positive effect on disease course.93,94 Sinemet was recently reported as the most commonly administered drug among more than 8,000 patients followed longitudinally in the National Parkinson Foundation Quality Improvement Initiative study.75 Expert practitioners reporting in this database utilized levodopa more than any other drug. These expert investigators actually used levodopa (Sinemet and Madopar) more and not less as Parkinson's disease progressed.

Recently an important study was published in The Lancet and included newly-diagnosed patients randomized to receive a dopamine agonist, a Monoamine Oxidase Inhibitor (MAO-I) or levodopa. The primary outcome was the mobility dimension on the Parkinson's disease questionnaire (PDQ-39) quality-of-life scale. There were 1,620 patients randomized, and the three-year follow-up revealed that the PDQ-39 mobility scores were better in the levodopa group as compared to the other two groups. Follow-up at seven years revealed levodopa was the best overall therapy. There was a small difference favoring initial therapy with the MAO-Is when this drug was compared to a dopamine agonist. The treatment-related side effects were overall less in the levodopa group.95,96

Over the past two decades, the trendy phenomenon referred to as "levodopa phobia" (intentionally avoiding prescriptions for levodopa) has impeded the best clinical care for many Parkinson's disease patients.89 An accompanying editorial to the recent article in The Lancet pointed out that levodopa phobia and the favoring of dopamine agonist therapy were primarily driven by aggressive pharmaceutical marketing.95 The Lancet study revealed that all three therapies should potentially be considered, but that ultimately the choice of drugs should be tailored to the patient. Patient-rated mobility favored initial levodopa therapy.

What this adds up to for patients is that Sinemet and Madopar should be considered safe and effective as initial treatments for Parkinson's disease. The doses and intervals should be frequently adjusted by an experienced neurologist or practitioner to maximize benefits and to tailor to individual symptoms. Patients and families should keep in perspective that the talk about levodopa being toxic and accelerating disease progression (levodopa phobia) can prove to be a major distractor to good care practices. Precious minutes in the doctor-patient relationship should not be wasted on these claims. Prescribers should not avoid levodopa or intentionally underdose this critical therapy, especially in patients with treatable symptoms. Critics of Sinemet and Madopar will need to bring forward much stronger human data if they wish to change clinical practice. In the meantime, we need to serve our patients by sharing with them the weight of the evidence which strongly supports that levodopa replacement therapy is not toxic, does not accelerate Parkinson's disease progression and can be used safely as initial therapy.97

What are the currently available treatments for Parkinson's disease beyond levodopa replacement?

Dopamine Agonists (tickle a few dopamine receptors in the brain)

- Mirapex (pramipexole)
- Requip (ropinirole)
- Neupro (rotigotine transdermal - the patch)

Quick Acting Dopamine agonist by injection under the Skin

- Apokyn (apomorphine)

Monoamine Oxidase B Inhibitors (stop the breakdown of dopamine and makeit more available)

- Zelapar (zydis selegiline)
- Azilect (rasagiline)

- Selegiline (generic)

Anticholinergics (block the cholinergic receptor in the brain)

- Trihexyphenidyl (Artane)
- Benztropine (Cogentin)
- Biperiden (Akineton)
- Orphenadrine (Disipal)
- Procyclidine (Kemadrin)

Antiviral therapy that works on many brain receptors including dopamine and glutamate

- Symmetrel (amantadine)

Dopamine Extenders (block the breakdown of dopamine)

- Comtan (entacapone)
- Tasmar (tolcapone)

Take Home Points

- Rytary is a new extended release dopamine formulation that may help some patients, especially those trying to maintain three times a day dosing of their medications.
- Dopamine agonists have been associated with a worse side effect profile compared to Sinemet, and they are highly associated with impulse control disorders.
- The patch formulation (Rotigotine) may be associated with less impulse control disorders.
- The COMT inhibitors like Stalevo can precipitate and worsen dyskinesia, though there is hope newer formulation such as Opicapone will be better options.

- MAO-B inhibitors are good symptomatic options, and the best evidence exists for Rasagiline, but Selegiline has also been shown effective, though it does have an amphetamine metabolite.
- There is considerable debate as to whether the 1mg dose of Rasagiline may be slightly neuroprotective.
- Medication should be started when a patient is symptomatic and also when symptoms are affecting quality of life or threatening injury.

Chapter 4

Marijuana and Synthetic Cannabinoids

"It really puzzles me to see marijuana connected with narcotics ... dope and all that crap. It's a thousand times better than whiskey. It is an assistant and a friend."

–Louis Armstrong

THERE HAS BEEN a recent and evolving media blitz concerning the potential use of medical marijuana (tetrahydrocannabinol, THC) in Parkinson's disease patients. All of the attention to marijuana has been largely a result of multiple states passing legislation to legalize and regulate the drug. The ultimate goal of this activity is to make marijuana available for select and appropriate medical diagnoses. Recent advocates for this position, including Sanjay Gupta from CNN, have been gaining unprecedented momentum.

There are several cannabinoid receptors in the brain. CB1 receptors are common in the regions of the brain most important to Parkinson's disease. CB2 receptors, in contrast, seem to be more important for immunity to disease, but these receptors also are present in the brain. CB2 receptors could be important in regulating Parkinson's disease symptoms such as dyskinesia. The many different formulations of marijuana and synthetic versions can be tweaked to affect different receptor classes and also can be changed to curb or enhance euphoria and other drug effects. Additionally, cannabidiol (CBD) which is a cannabis constituent may have therapeutic value with a better adverse effect profile. It is important to keep in mind that there are potential drugs available that can stimulate the cannabinoid receptor (agonists) and those that can block it (antagonists). Interestingly, sometimes the blocker drugs in low dose actually stimulate the cannabinoid receptors.

A recent report from the guideline development subcommittee of the American Academy of Neurology (AAN) tackled the evidence base supporting the use of marijuana for neurological disorders. Spasticity, central pain syndromes and bladder dysfunction were improved by marijuana. The few available studies have revealed that marijuana was not helpful in Parkinson's disease-related tremor or levodopa-induced dyskinesia. The report was careful to outline the risks and benefits of medical marijuana, and it recommended education and counseling for anyone considering this option. The risk of serious psychopathologic effects (hallucinations, etc.) was cited at one percent.98

In addition to the AAN report, there have been a few recent papers supporting the use of marijuana for specific Parkinson's disease symptoms, such as motor, mood, quality of life and sleep; however, all of these papers have suffered from methodological issues such as small numbers of patients and lack of a control group. In a 2004 issue of the Movement Disorders journal, a survey by Katerina Venderova was published regarding Parkinson's disease patients using marijuana (cannabis). She reported that "39 patients (45.9%) described mild or substantial alleviation of their Parkinson's disease symptoms in general, 26 (30.6%) showed improvement of rest tremor, 38 (44.7%) had improvement in bradykinesia, 32 (37.7%) had alleviation of muscle rigidity, and 12 (14.1%) had improvement of L-dopa-induced dyskinesia. Only 4 patients in this survey (4.7%) reported that cannabis actually worsened their symptoms. Patients using cannabis for at least 3 months reported significantly more alleviation of their Parkinson's disease symptoms in general."99 Like Venderova, who conducted her survey in Prague, we have collected anecdotes from Parkinson's disease patients who have phoned us at the free National Parkinson Foundation hotline (1-800-4PD-INFO), and we have heard personal experiences and positive stories supportive of the use of marijuana in Parkinson's disease. Collectively, the problem with all of these types of personal reports has been the lack of scientific rigor necessary to truly understand the effects of marijuana on Parkinson's disease.

In a recent review in the New England Journal of Medicine, the National Institute on Drug Abuse (NIDA) Director Nora Volkow, M.D., carefully outlined the adverse health effects of marijuana use.100 In her article, Volkow pointed out that marijuana, which is thought of by much of the public as a completely harmless drug, can have serious adverse effects. She makes the following important points:

- In the U.S., marijuana is the most commonly used "illicit" drug.
- 12 percent of those 12 years or older used it in the past year.
- Smoking is the most common way people use marijuana, and this can harm the lungs.
- There are available edible forms including teas and foods.
- Approximately nine percent of users will become addicted, and there may be a withdrawal syndrome that can make quitting difficult for some users.
- Use in adolescence and early adulthood can contribute to worsening brain function, decreased connections between brain regions and a decrease in IQ.
- Heavy marijuana use can rarely lead to psychosis and hallucinations.
- Marijuana can reduce cognitive and can also worsen motor function.
- Your risk of a car accident doubles if you have recently smoked marijuana.
- The potency of the THC content in marijuana has increased from three to 12 percent in the last several decades, making accidental overdoses, especially with food products, much more common.
- The best evidence supporting marijuana use has been shown in glaucoma, nausea, the AIDS wasting syndrome, chronic pain, multiple sclerosis and epilepsy.

Scientifically, it is not crazy to think that marijuana may play some positive role in the alleviation of Parkinson's disease symptoms. There are cannabinoid (THC) receptors all over the brain, and these receptors seem to be concentrated in a region important to Parkinson's disease, commonly referred to as the basal ganglia. In fact, the globus pallidus and the substantia nigra pars reticulata, which are structures within the basal ganglia important to the generation of Parkinson's disease symptoms, are some of the most densely packed cannabinoid (THC) receptor areas in the human body. Therefore, it is not beyond reason to consider the possibility that a drug directed at these receptors might positively influence the symptoms of Parkinson's disease. Indeed, many drug companies remain interested in compounds influencing these receptors.101

What is the bottom line if you have Parkinson's disease and you are considering medical marijuana? Marijuana should never be thought of as a replacement for dopaminergic and other approved therapies for Parkinson's disease. Second, though most available large studies have not shown a marijuana benefit, that does not mean that there will not be a benefit. More research will be needed to understand which patients could benefit, which symptoms could be affected and how best to safely administer medical marijuana in Parkinson's disease, especially over the long-term. It may turn out that non-motor features such as depression, anxiety and pain respond best; however, before we jump to conclusions we should pursue careful studies to sort out all of the effects. Parkinson's disease patients living in states where marijuana has been legalized for medical use should be aware of the dangers outlined by Nora Volkow, particularly the effects on the lungs, the dangers of driving and accidental overdoses (particularly with food items).100 Finally, states will need to develop training programs for doctors and medical teams prescribing marijuana so that the Parkinson's disease patient on medical marijuana can be kept as safe as possible.102

Synthetic Cannabinoids

Patients need to be aware that since Woodstock there have been changes in the availability and the types of marijuana. The most important thing to be aware of is the burgeoning market for synthetic cannabinoids. A synthetic or manufactured version of marijuana may be similar to THC, but different elements of the structure can be altered. There are many formulations including those that can be smoked, eaten (powders) or sold as teas. Perhaps the most well known synthetic version of marijuana has been sold under the name Spice. Other common product names include Kronic, Northern Lights, K2, Zeus, Puff, Tai High, Aroma, K2, fake weed, Yucatan Fire, Skunk, Moon Rocks and Magic Dragon. Though Spice and other synthetic cannabinoids may be illegal in many states, manufacturers may skirt state and federal laws by replacing and manipulating chemicals in the synthetic version.

Experiences with synthetic versions of marijuana have not always been positive. There has been a recent surge of patients visiting emergency rooms after ingesting synthetic cannabinoids. Rapid heart rates, vomiting, agitation, confusion and hallucinations have all been reported. Poison control centers have also recently reported an uptick in synthetic cannabinoid toxicity. Additionally, there have been withdrawal and addiction symptoms reported with some formulations. Because of the current safety issues most expert practitioners discourage synthetic cannabinoids for Parkinson's disease, though there may be a brighter horizon in the future as more is learned.

A Change in Prescribing Guidelines for Marijuana?

Many people believe that to move the field forward and to understand and realize the potential benefits of medical marijuana, there will need to be a fundamental shift in philosophy on the drug. Benzi Kluger, a former fellow at University of Florida and now a movement disorders expert at the University of Colorado along with Joseph Jankovic at Baylor University, have suggested that a change in classification from Schedule I to Schedule IV or V in the DEA prescription guidelines "would not only improve access to medical marijuana but could facilitate development and conduct of clinical trials for cannabinoids." We will need to study both marijuana and synthetic cannabinoids to better understand their potential therapeutic uses in Parkinson's disease.100

Take Home Points:

- There is mounting evidence that marijuana may be useful for the treatment of Parkinson's disease symptoms.
- The fundamental issue in the field is that we do not yet know for which symptoms and for which Parkinson's disease patients medical marijuana may be helpful.
- Patients and families should beware of the potential adverse effects of marijuana: effect on the lungs, dangers of driving, and potential for accidental overdoses (particularly with food items).
- Patients and families should be cautious about using synthetic cannabinoids until we define which formulations are safe and effective.
- A change in prescribing guidelines may help us to move the field forward.

CHAPTER 5

New Drugs for Hallucinations, Sleep, Constipation and Dizziness

I respectfully decline the invitation to join your hallucination.

-Scott Adams

Hallucinations

WHEN WE RECENTLY examined the topics that were most searched for (i.e. hit) on our website, we were not surprised to discover that treatment of psychosis and hallucinations in Parkinson's disease topped the list. There has been a critical, unmet need for development of better drugs to address hallucinations and psychosis in the setting of Parkinson's disease. We have learned over many years that typical high potency neuroleptic antipsychotic drugs (e.g. Haldol, Olanzapine) may improve hallucinations but do so at the cost of worsening Parkinson's disease motor symptoms (rigidity, slowness and walking). We have changed our treatment strategy to address hallucinations in Parkinson's disease by using agents that will not worsen the common motor symptoms (stiffness, slowness, walking). We routinely choose quetiapine (Seroquel) or clozapine (Clozaril) instead of the classical dopamine blocking drugs. There are, however, shortcomings with these two drugs. Quetiapine has not been shown effective across several randomized Parkinson's disease clinical trials, but many Parkinson experts believe it is moderately helpful particularly in the setting of mild hallucinations. Clozapine has been shown to be highly efficacious, but it requires weekly blood monitoring to check for a potentially life-threatening side effect called agranulocytosis, where the drug attacks the bone marrow. The inconvenience and discomfort of blood draws have limited the penetration of this therapy.103-105 Pimavanserin is a new drug that works primarily on the serotonin receptor. It does not block the dopamine receptor and does not worsen the Parkinson's disease motor symptoms.33,106-112 Here are some tips about what you need to know about Pimavanserin for treatment of Parkinson's disease related psychosis.

- Though classically we think about the dopamine receptor in Parkinson's disease as underpinning psychosis symptoms, serotonin has also been implicated.
- Lysergic acid diethylamide and phencyclidine (PCP) stimulate 5-HT2A serotonin type of receptors. Stimulation of these receptors may lead to hallucinations.
- Most available antipsychotic drugs block the 5HT2A receptor and the D2 dopamine receptor.
- It is possible that the 5HT2A blocking mechanisms of newer antipsychotics may underpin their benefit and may do so with a lower side effect portfolio (leaving out the D2 blocking effects).
- Pimavanserin is a 5HT2A inverse agonist. It binds to the same receptor as an agonist; an agonist would stimulate the receptor, but an inverse agonist would do the opposite and reduce stimulation below basal levels for the serotonin brain receptor.
- Pimavanserin is thought to have few or no motor side effects (e.g. tardive dyskinesia, parkinsonism).
- The emerging safety profile has shown it is potentially superior to other available antipsychotics.
- There is one Phase III trial that has shown benefit.

It is possible that Pimavanserin will be another great alternative for some patients with Parkinson's disease, especially since it does not worsen motor symptoms, but more data will be needed. One wonders if in severe cases of psychosis, Pimavanserin could be added to seroquel or to clozaril to improve treatment of difficult to control hallucinations. 33,106-112

Patients should keep in mind that there are a few general rules that most experts will employ when treating psychosis. First, practitioners will discontinue or reduce dosages of many hallucination and psychosis triggering medications (amantadine, MAO-B inhibitors, anticholinergics, entacapone, and dopamine agonists). Sometimes, patients can be maintained on Sinemet-only (carbidopa/levodopa) regimens or can reduce Sinemet dose and increase the frequency of dose administrations. When these strategies don't work, many PD experts turn to quetipine, clozapine and possibly Pimavanserin (NUPLAZID) pending FDA approval.113 The FDA has placed a black box warning on clozapine because of the risk of agranulocystosis (loss of white blood cells which are important for immunity) and this warning calls for weekly monitoring of blood counts. Quetiapine has a FDA box warning because of an increased mortality when used in elderly patients with dementia and psychosis. Despite these warnings most experts believe that Clozapine and Quetiapine are the safest hallucination drugs for use in Parkinson's disease patients. We will have to wait for the safety profile of Pimavanserin to emerge, but early testing has revealed that it could be safer than the alternatives.

Sleep and Melatonin: Light is Better than the Pill

Many investigators have focused on melatonin as an important chemical in the human sleep-wake circadian rhythm. Melatonin is manufactured in the center of the brain in a structure called the pineal gland. René Descartes referred to the pineal gland as the "seat of the soul." Melatonin from the pineal gland can trigger sleepiness and can also lower body temperature. The manufacture of melatonin is disrupted by exposure to light. Researchers have postulated that intervening in the melatonin pathways by exposing Parkinson's disease patients to bright light could have a therapeutic benefit.

Aleksander Videnovic and colleagues at the National Parkinson Foundation Center of Excellence at Harvard University recently explored blood melatonin tests that were sampled over 24 hours.114,115 The tests were designed to uncover some of the mysteries of fatigue and the sleep-wake disturbances in Parkinson's disease. The researchers studied 20 Parkinson's patients and 20 control patients without Parkinson's. Melatonin blood levels were checked every 30 minutes for 24 straight hours. Parkinson's patients failed to secrete melatonin in a normal pattern. Parkinson's disease patients in the study who suffered from excessive daytime sleepiness or fatigue had more dysfunction in the patterns of melatonin than those without excessive daytime sleepiness or fatigue. How long a patient had Parkinson's disease, how severe their motor symptoms were and what medications they were taking were not related to the circadian rhythm. The authors postulated that sleep-wake circadian function could be improved by timed exposure to bright light and also potentially exercise. There have been several other small studies that have also suggested Parkinson's disease motor symptoms, as well as non-motor symptoms, may improve with light therapy.

At the 66th Annual Meeting of the American Academy of Neurology (2014), Videnovic and colleagues presented another study on the preliminary results of light therapy for excessive daytime sleepiness or fatigue. There were 30 patients included with an average duration of disease of approximately seven years. The study intervention was bright light therapy (5000 lux) or dim red-light therapy (300 lux) delivered for two hours a day for 14 days. The results did not reveal a difference between the groups, but a closer look at the scores in this small study revealed that the Epworth Sleepiness Scale improved by 2.3 points in the dim red light group, and 4.3 points in the bright light therapy group. Though these results were not robust, they suggested at least the tantalizing possibility that light therapy could be optimized for better results in Parkinson's disease. Some researchers have suggested that better penetrance of light therapy could be delivered through other techniques, including deep brain electrodes, but this remains highly investigational and has only been attempted in animals.

If melatonin release is blocked by exposure to light, and if exposing patients to light may improve Parkinson's disease symptoms, why would patients intentionally take melatonin? Melatonin (N-acetyl-5-methoxy-tryptamine) is an antioxidant. Neurodegenerative disorders such as Parkinson's disease have been linked to oxidative damage and free radical generation, and some people believe that melatonin may help in blocking neurodegeneration. However, there are no human studies to support the notion that melatonin slows or blocks neurodegeneration. Some patients also use melatonin for sleep issues; though again there are no large well-controlled studies to support this notion, and in many cases reports have surfaced that melatonin replacement may actually worsen sleep in Parkinson's disease. I have personally listened to the stories from several of my own patients who have tried melatonin and reported worsening in sleep. If you decide to try melatonin (which is over the counter) for sleep, you should do it under the guidance of a physician. Until more data is published, we cannot make a recommendation as to the usefulness of melatonin replacement for sleep issues.

The bottom line is there is accumulating evidence that melatonin is important to sleep and to excessive daytime sleepiness in Parkinson's disease. Melatonin can possibly be powerfully modulated by light therapy and also exercise. Melatonin pills may not be the answer for many patients with Parkinson's disease and could potentially worsen symptoms. More research will be needed to clarify how shining a light on Parkinson's disease may provide a new option for patients, especially those with excessive daytime sleepiness.116

Constipation

One of the most common questions we receive on the "Ask the Doctor" National Parkinson Foundation forum is how best to address constipation. This symptom is both common and disabling in Parkinson's disease, and there is a critical need for newer and better approaches.

Under-recognized and undertreated, constipation affects the majority of Parkinson's disease sufferers. Bill Ondo and colleagues from the University of

Michael S Okun MD

Texas evaluated the efficacy and tolerability of lubiprostone (Amitiza) as a treatment for constipation. Ondo utilized a double-blind, randomized and controlled study. Doses were titrated over two weeks, and patients were followed for four weeks. Fifty-four subjects received lubiprostone or a placebo drug therapy. The results revealed a "marked or very marked clinical global improvement in 16 of 25 (64.0%) subjects versus 5 of 27 (18.5%) receiving placebo (p < 0.001)." Constipation rating scales and stool diaries improved on Amitiza. The adverse event profile was excellent, and loose stools were the most common individual patient complaint.117,118

The original 1817 essay describing Parkinson disease actually included constipation as an important patient issue.119 Almost 200 years later, our patients still suffer with this issue. We now recognize that it takes the stomach longer to empty, and it also takes longer for food to move through the intestines in Parkinson's disease. Muscles and nerves within the gastrointestinal tract in Parkinson's disease are affected by the degenerative process, and protein deposits called Lewy bodies have been discovered in the intestines of these patients. Lewy bodies are also found in the brains of Parkinson's disease patients, and their presence in the intestines infers constipation is likely a core symptom of Parkinson's disease.

The drug lubiprostone acts by turning on chloride channels in the mucosa of the gastrointestinal tract. It enhances fluid secretion and improves the overall movement of the stomach and intestines. Importantly, it does not affect blood electrolytes such as sodium and potassium, making it potentially a very safe treatment.

Common treatment approaches for constipation in Parkinson's disease have included:

- Optimization of Parkinson's drugs
- Polyethylene glycol
- Lactulose
- Sorbitol

54

- Fiber supplements
- Six to eight glasses of plain water a day
- Vigorous daily exercise
- Stool softeners
- Enemas

*It is important to treat constipation more aggressively if 2-3 days pass without a bowel movement. You should contact your physician and try to avoid a hospitalization. Many patients will use enemas to avoid hospitalization and manual disimpaction.

Lubriprostone (Amitiza) is a promising advance in the care of the Parkinson's disease patient. Though it may not work for every sufferer, it should be considered a potential option. We recommend that patients employ a comprehensive plan to address constipation. Over the years, we have found the use of many of the possible therapies (listed above and often in combination), to be extremely helpful remedies. Future studies of Lubriprostone will need to be longer than four weeks and should include more information of the type of Parkinson's disease patient most likely to benefit.

A new drug called Ghrelin RM-131 (Rhythm Pharmaceuticals) is currently in trial. It works on an important nerve called the vagus nerve. Ghrelin stimulates the stomach and intestines and blocks insulin release from the pancreas. A clinical trial in Parkinson's disease patients is currently underway.120-122

Recently, Drs. Jose Barboza, Baharak Moshiree and I reviewed the up-and-coming treatments for constipation in Parkinson's disease and two other drugs drew our attention.

Linaclotide is FDA approved for the treatment of chronic constipation and irritable bowel syndrome with constipation; however, it has not been studied in patients with Parkinson's disease. This newer medication promotes the generation of cyclic guanosine monophosphate that secretes chloride and bicarbonate into the intestinal lumen, increasing luminal fluid secretion and accelerating intestinal transit. Linaclotide at 145 or 290 mcg/day led to more complete spontaneous bowel movements (SBM) per week compared to placebo in a double-blind RCT in 1,276 patients for up to 12 weeks. Diarrhea was the most common adverse event. Although linaclotide has not been tested in Parkinson's disease, it has shown to be efficacious in treating constipation in general, and may be used in Parkinson's disease if other options have been unsuccessful. Moreover, linaclotide also directly inhibits pain by acting on the C-fibres in the colon and may prove beneficial in patients with abdominal pain.

The GI tract is host to 95 percent of the body's serotonin, and the activation of these receptors stimulates the peristaltic reflex, enhances intestinal secretions and reduces visceral hypersensitivity, all of which may help in treatment of constipation. Mosapride and prucalopride are used to treat chronic constipation; however, they are not yet FDA approved. Mosapride is available in Asia and South America, and prucalopride is available in Canada and Europe. Although not extensively evaluated in Parkinson's disease and constipation, a small open-label trial from Japan evaluated mosapride 15mg daily in 14 patients (seven with Parkinson's disease and seven with multiple system atrophy). Zhi Liu and colleagues found subjective improvements in bowel frequency and defecation in patients with Parkinson's disease. Due to the lack of an appropriate study design with mosapride, we do not recommend using this agent in patients with Parkinson's disease until further larger trials can be completed. Although both the use of mosapride and prucalopride appear to be safe in the general population, they are currently lacking evidence in the Parkinson's disease population.

A novel mechanism, ileal sodium/bile acid co-transporter (IBAT) modulator, is being investigated for the treatment of constipation. Elobixibat is a minimally-absorbed IBAT that partially inhibits the ileal bile acid transporter. It has been shown to increase fluid secretion and motility by modulating bile acid synthesis and enterohepatic circulation resulting ultimately in the increased delivery of bile acid to the colon. A dose-finding study revealed that elobixibat significantly increased the number of bowel movements per week compared to placebo in patients with chronic constipation. Large multi-center phase III trials are underway to determine the efficacy and safety elobixibat when administered over 26 weeks. The section on newer constipation treatments is drawn from unpublished expert opinion work from Drs. Barboza, Moshiree and Okun.123

Finally, one recently appreciated phenomenon is dyssynergic defecation. This issue occurs when there is an inability, of the pelvic floor muscles to relax during defecation. This can be a cause for constipation in Parkinson's disease and some authors have suggested that biofeedback could be a treatment option.

Dizziness and Passing Out

There may be good news for Parkinson's disease patients suffering from low blood pressure, dizziness and passing out (syncope) as a new drug recently received FDA approval: Droxidopa, now labeled Northera. Over many years of clinical practice, I have seen Parkinson's disease patients visit the emergency room or clinic because of dizziness and/or passing out. In most cases, the obligatory cardiac evaluation does not uncover an underlying factor explaining the symptom. Many patients are referred to a vestibular physical therapist (someone who specializes in eye movement and gait stabilization) to fix the vertigo; however, this approach is useful for only a few patients. Most patients actually have orthostatic hypotension which can be a manifestation of Parkinson's disease, and this common manifestation can be made worse by Parkinson's medications.

Orthostatic hypotension is common in Parkinson's disease and affects fifteen to 50 percent of patients. It has been defined as a drop in systolic blood pressure of greater than 20 mmHg or a decrease in diastolic blood pressure of greater than 10mmHg within three minutes of changing to a standing position. Joseph Jankovic and colleagues at the Baylor National Parkinson Foundation Center of Excellence in Houston, TX recently published information about orthostatic hypotension in a large series of Parkinson's disease patients. Jankovic reviewed the records of 1,318 patients and found that symptomatic orthostatic hypotension occurred in "81% of patients with multiple system atrophy, in 18%

of Parkinson's disease, and in 19% with non-multiple system atrophy (MSA), a form of atypical parkinsonism." Jankovic taught us that orthostatic hypotension occurred in older patients with more advanced Parkinson's disease and those with longer disease durations.124-126

When orthostatic hypotension is verified, patients should consider reducing or eliminating the medications that contribute to the problem, including antihypertensive medications. I always say that the one fringe benefit of a diagnosis of Parkinson's disease may be retiring your blood pressure pills.

Dopaminergic medications (particularly the dopamine agonists) may worsen orthostatic hypotension. Non-pharmacologic strategies that may improve orthostatic symptoms include increasing fluid intake, increasing dietary salt and caffeine and using tight, thigh-high support stockings to prevent pooling of blood below the waist. Purchasing a hospital bed or raising the head of a normal bed 10 to 30 degrees may improve the standing blood pressure when it is performed on a regular basis over several weeks. If needed, drugs to raise blood pressure may be used.127-129 Fludrocortisone and midodrine are the most common drugs used for treatment of orthostasis in Parkinson's disease, and these strategies work best with concomitant increases hydration.125 Some practitioners add drugs like Mestinon, which has been used for myasthenia gravis.

The newest medication that has been recently FDA approved is called droxidopa (Northera), L-threo-3,4,-dihydroxyphenylserine. This drug is a pro-drug of norepinephrine. The drug has shown promise in multiple system atrophy (MSA) and in cases of pure autonomic failure. Several recent studies report its usefulness in Parkinson's disease. We do not possess enough data on droxidopa to know if it will be effective for the subset of Parkinson's disease patients who are suffering with low blood pressure symptoms and who have not discovered relief with the available alternatives and medications. The studies leading to the approval of droxidopa were only conducted for two weeks, and the approval was offered as part of the FDA's new accelerated process. The one side effect of Northera (droxipdopa) that is potentially most worrisome is skyrocketing blood pressure when laying down (supine hypertension), but this is also an issue with other available drugs.127,128,130-133

The bottom line for Parkinson's disease patients who are passing out (syncope), or getting dizzy, especially when standing up or when changing positions, is that this may be your Parkinson's disease, your Parkinson's disease medications or potentially both. Consult your doctor immediately, and have your blood pressure taken while lying down, sitting and also standing. There are many effective strategies that may improve your quality of life, and these may prevent dizziness and passing out. We hope the new drug Northera will provide many of our PD patients with another option for orthostatic hypotension.134

Take Home Points:

- Hallucinations, even when mild, can present both safety and quality of life issues.
- Treatment with quetiapine and clozapine have been the best drug approaches as these two medications do not worsen motor symptoms of Parkinson's disease.
- A new medication that works on the serotonin system called Pimavanserin may be an option for some patients with hallucinations.
- Melatonin may worsen sleep in some Parkinson's disease patients.
- Light therapy is a promising approach to sleep and non-motor symptoms.
- Constipation is important to address in Parkinson's disease, and Lubriprostone and other new drugs may be helpful.
- There may be benefit of Linaclotide for abdominal pain in Parkinson's disease, but studies are needed.
- There is a new drug available for orthostatic hypotension (dizziness and passing out) called Northera.

CHAPTER 6

Therapies While Hospitalized and Avoiding Hospitalization

"The very first requirement in a hospital is that it should do the sick no harm."

-Florence Nightingale

VINCENT LOW AND colleagues in Great Britain recently examined hospital admission data from England's Hospital Episodes Statistics (HES) database. The investigators accessed 324,055 Parkinson's disease admissions. These admissions amounted to nearly one billion dollars in expenses. Pneumonias, urinary tract infections and hip fractures occurred two times more frequently in Parkinson's disease patients. Parkinson's disease patients were more likely to have extended hospital stays and to die in the hospital when compared to their peers.135 Rob Skelly and colleagues recently surveyed practitioners across Britain and discovered that "care for Parkinson's in-patients was not highly rated by U.K. Parkinson's clinicians."136,137

Many years ago in the United States, we became alarmed at the number of reports we were receiving from patients regarding negative experiences in the hospital. We decided to investigate these issues by utilizing the international network of National Parkinson Foundation Centers of Excellence.138,139 What we discovered from this effort was startling. This chapter was one of the most useful and cited work from our previous book, "Parkinson's Treatment: 10 Secrets to a Happier Life."6 and we have included it and updated the contents. I remind patients that breakthroughs in research include care as well as novel drugs and devices. This is an important update.

Hospitalization in Parkinson's Disease

Our research group, along with the National Parkinson Foundation team, published a series of five papers that aimed to identify and suggest improvements in care for the hospitalized Parkinson's disease patient. In the first paper, we aimed to review the literature and identify practice gaps in the management of the hospitalized Parkinson's disease patient.138 We were interested in this general question of hospitalization, as many experts had cited that patients with Parkinson's disease were typically admitted to hospitals at higher rates and frequently had longer hospital stays when compared to the general population. Our working group reviewed publications drawn from the previous 40 years. Most papers cited motor disturbances to be a causal factor in the higher rates of admissions and complications.

However, other conditions were commonly recorded as the primary reason for hospitalization. These included motor complications, reduced mobility, lack of medication compliance, inappropriate use of neuroleptics (dopamine blocking drugs), falls, fractures, pneumonia and other serious medical problems. There were many relevant issues identified and many were preventable. Most issues could be improved. Medications, dosages and specific dosage schedules were critical elements to the success of Parkinson's disease patients in the hospital, but it was clear that most hospital staff members were completely unaware of the factors that may torpedo a successful hospitalization.138

Hospital staff training regarding medications and medication management was universally deficient, and there was little in the literature to suggest that early mobility and prevention of aspiration pneumonia were critical, despite the known statistic that it was the number one killer in Parkinson's disease. We concluded that educational programs, recommendations and guidelines were all desperately needed and that these guidelines would likely save lives, provide a cost savings to the health care system and improve outcomes.

Management in the Hospital

In the second paper, we explored current practices and opinions on the management of the Parkinson's disease (PD) patient in the hospital by utilizing our network of 54 National Parkinson Foundation (NPF) Centers worldwide.140 We had each of our centers complete an online survey regarding hospitalization of Parkinson's disease patients. These centers were among an elite group of care facilities in the world, and 43 of them carried the prestigious and difficult to obtain Center of Excellence designation. Many centers reported grave concern about the quality of Parkinson's disease-specific care that was provided to their patients when hospitalized. The biggest concerns included adherence to the patient's outpatient medication schedule and the lack of understanding and appreciation by hospital staff of the medications that could worsen Parkinson's disease.

Surprisingly, few NPF Centers of Excellence had an existing policy within their primary hospital that facilitated immediate notification of the Parkinson's doctor if their patient was admitted to the hospital. Shockingly, notification of hospitalization typically was accomplished directly from the patient or a family member. About one-third of centers reported not finding out about a patient being hospitalized until a routine clinic visit following discharge. These visits could occur as far out as many months following discharge. Quick access to outpatient care was lacking across most centers. Elective surgery, falls, fractures, infections and confusion were all identified as common reasons for hospitalization.

We concluded that there was a need for involvement of a Parkinson's disease specialist or at least a neurologist when patients were admitted to the hospital. Education of hospital staff and clinicians regarding the management of Parkinson's disease, complications and medications to avoid was a critically unaddressed issue. Most importantly, outpatient access should be improved to prevent unnecessary hospitalizations.

Risk Factors for Hospitalization

In the third and most important paper, we sought to identify risk factors for hospitalization (emergency room visits or admissions) among Parkinson's disease patients followed in our National Parkinson Foundation Quality Improvement Initiative.139 The initiative was modeled after a similar effort put together by Gerry O'Connor at the Dartmouth Health Outcomes Center. O'Connor had a crazy but practical idea. He would collect one page of data once a year on all cystic fibrosis patients and use the data to benchmark how centers were doing. This procedure promoted best practices. Most leading scientists viewed this approach as a waste of time, energy and money. The registry, however, paid big dividends, and based on issues identified across the network of cystic fibrosis centers nationwide, the average age a cystic fibrosis patient now lives is 10 years longer (from approximately 28 to 38 years of age).

Joyce Oberdorf, CEO of the National Parkinson Foundation, hired O'Connor to replicate the same program but to work with our experts to transform and grow the fundamental idea into the Parkinson's disease field. Oberdorf hired a young talent and data whiz from Harvard and later Cornell University named Peter Schmidt. Schmidt was hungry to help people after a successful career as an investment banker. He, along with Andy Siderowf from the University of Pennsylvania, Mark Guttman from Markham in Toronto, and John Nutt from the University of Oregon, helped to organize a group of skeptical clinician-scientists into the National Parkinson Foundation Quality Improvement Study.75

The first cut of the data from the initiative yielded 3,060 patients, and shockingly, 1,016 (33 percent) had a hospitalization in the first year. Of those, 49 percent had a readmission in the second year. Those who were not hospitalized the first year of the study had a 25 percent risk of a new hospitalization in the second year.

The data from the study was assembled by our young Australian fellow, Anhar Hassan, who is now on faculty at the Mayo Clinic in Rochester, Minnesota. The surprising wake-up call was that Parkinson's disease patients had very high rates of hospitalization (ER visits or admissions) and that these hospitalizations were associated with advanced disease, more co-morbid conditions (e.g. hypertension, heart disease, lung issues, etc.), and a longer time to rise from a chair, walk 10 meters and return to the chair (referred to as a Timed Up and Go Test). Quality of life was worse for those hospitalized, and not surprisingly, there was a higher burden on the caregiver. Just as in O'Connor's study of cystic fibrosis, some centers performed better than others suggesting that there may be more optimal approaches to improve care and to prevent hospitalization.

We have now recently presented a fourth paper on the rate of hospital encounters over a five-year period. We aimed to create a profile for patients with and without frequent encounters and to identify any associated and potentially modifiable factors. Our fellow from Tehran, Leili Shahgholi Ghahfarkhi examined 7,507 patients and presented the data at the 2015 American Academy of Neurology meeting in Washington, D.C.141 The rate of hospital encounters was 25.6 percent, 32.8 percent, 34.9 percent, 34 .2 percent and 38.5 percent for years one through five, respectively. We learned that Parkinson's disease patients had a high risk for hospitalization, and the risk increased slightly in subsequent years. Co-morbidities, disease stage, mobility, prior DBS, levodopa usage and caregiver strain were all identified as risk factors associated with hospitalization or re-hospitalization.

Finally, we were also interested in examining our own experience at the University of Florida and particularly in looking at details that may impact the actual experience of the hospitalized Parkinson's disease patient. Danny Martinez, our fellow at the time, from Monterrey, Mexico, reviewed 212 Parkinson's disease subjects admitted to our hospital.142 Martinez is now the NPF's "Ask the Spanish Doctor" and has translated this book and the "10 Secrets" book into Spanish. Interestingly, Parkinson's disease patients who had delayed administration or missed at least one dose stayed longer in the hospital. Twenty-three percent of Parkinson's patients took dopamine-blocking agents, and these dose administrations had the potential to worsen Parkinson's disease symptoms. These drugs led to an increased length of stay (8.2 days vs. 3.6 days).

Drugs to Avoid in Parkinson's Disease

Whether in or out of the hospital, it is important to understand what drugs should be avoided in Parkinson's disease patients. A good friend of mine and very experienced senior neurologist Ed Steinmetz from Ft. Myers, Fla., pointed out to me a list of such drugs recently published in the Public Citizen newsletter (http://www.citizen.org). The approach was to list every drug associated with a single confirmed or unconfirmed symptom of Parkinson's disease or parkinsonism.

Patients and family members confronted with a simple "drug list" approach may falsely conclude that most medicines are bad for Parkinson's disease and even worse, that any medicine may cause parkinsonism. This concept is, in general, incorrect. Although the approach is well meaning, it is in need of a major revision as Parkinson's disease is too complex to summarize by simple lists.

It is well known that drugs that block dopamine worsen Parkinson's disease, whereas dopamine replacement therapies (e.g. carbidopa/levodopa, Sinemet, dopamine agonists) may improve symptoms. One of the big issues facing many Parkinson's disease patients is psychosis (e.g. hallucinations, illusions and behavioral changes such as paranoia). How does one concomitantly administer dopamine replacement therapy, which may in some cases induce psychosis, while at the same time administer dopamine-blocker drugs aimed at alleviating psychosis? Will the drugs cancel each other out?

There are two dopamine blockers that will, in general, not cancel out dopamine replacement, therefore not appreciably worsen Parkinson's disease. One is Quetiapine (Seroquel) and the other is Clozapine (Clozaril). Clozapine is the more powerful of the two drugs, but it requires weekly blood monitoring. Other classical dopamine blocking drugs, also referred to as neuroleptics (e.g. Haldol), worsen Parkinson's disease. Every Parkinson's disease patient and doctor should be aware of these two drugs that are the preferred treatment for psychosis occurring inside or outside of the hospital.

Patients may not be aware that some common drugs used for conditions such as headache or gastrointestinal dysmotility may also block dopamine and concomitantly worsen Parkinson's disease or alternatively result in parkinsonism (Parkinson's-like symptoms). These drugs include Prochlorperazine (Compazine), Promethazine (Phenergan) and Metoclopramide (Reglan). They drugs should be avoided. Also, drugs that deplete dopamine, such as reserpine and tetrabenazine, may worsen Parkinson's disease and should be avoided in most cases. Substitute drugs that do not result in worsening can be utilized, and these include Ondansetron (Zofran) for nausea and erythromycin, azithromycin or domperidone for gastrointestinal motility. Domperidone is not available in the U.S. but can sometimes be compounded by specialty pharmacies upon request. The availability of compounded drugs in the U.S. is unfortunately waning in light of the contamination issues that recently led to an outbreak of meningitis.

Antidepressants, anxiolytics, mood stabilizers, thyroid replacement drugs and antihypertensives are generally safe and do not worsen Parkinson's disease. They appear commonly on lists, including those provided by the Public Citizen, but don't be misled. Occasionally, there are reactions that lead to worsening of Parkinson's disease, but these are very rare occurrences. The bigger issue is drug-drug interactions. The most commonly encountered drug-drug interaction in Parkinson's disease is mixing a MAO-B Inhibitor (Selegline, Rasagiline, Azilect, Zelapar, Selegiline Hydrochloride dissolvable) with a pain medicine such as Meperidine (Demerol).

Also, MAO-A Inhibitors (e.g. Pirlindole) should not be taken with antidepressants. It should be kept in mind that in rare instances, mixing an antidepressant with another class of drugs can in select cases result in a serotonin syndrome (increased heart rate, tremor, sweating, big pupils, twitchy muscles and hyperactive reflexes). MAO-Bs, in almost all cases, are safe to take concomitantly with antidepressants, though many pharmacists will question the potential interaction and refuse to fill prescriptions. A refusal to fill a prescription should be challenged by your doctor.

The list approach to the worst pills in Parkinson's disease and parkinsonism is in need of a critical reappraisal. A more refined approach would take into consideration the complexities of Parkinson's disease and appreciate that with physician guidance and few exceptions, most drugs can be safely and effectively administered in Parkinson's disease and parkinsonism. This approach should be inclusive of many of the over-the-counter pills marked "not for use in Parkinson's disease."143

"Aware in Care" Campaign

NPF used the information on hospitalization and worst drugs in Parkinson's disease to fuel an effort to assist hospitalized patients. The problem NPF encountered was that patients could not depend on every hospital and every hospital employee worldwide to understand what to do and what not to do in Parkinson's disease management. The idea was to create a kit much like the bag that is packed and ready for a last trimester pregnant woman, a kit that has everything you need to survive the hospitalization.

The kit is large enough to pack your medications and also includes several critical elements:

1- A hospital action plan that provides tips on how to prepare for the next hospital visit
2- A Parkinson's disease identification bracelet
3- A medical alert card
4- A medication form to keep a list of active medications
5- A Parkinson's disease fact sheet to hand to the hospital staff and to be placed in your chart
6- "I have Parkinson's disease" reminder slips to educate hospital staff

7-   A thank you card for the staff member who provided the highest-quality Parkinson's care

The kit reinforces the simple platform that Parkinson's disease patients require their medications on time, every time and that many common drugs used in the hospital will worsen Parkinson's disease.

Secrets that can make your hospital stays shorter and potentially improve your condition include:

- Preventable errors in the hospital save lives.
- You and your family should assume the role of the "advocate."
- You and your family must educate all staff and physicians you contact.
- You will need to re-emphasize that Parkinson's disease patients require medications on time, every time.
- You will need to educate that Parkinson's disease symptoms worsen with sleep deprivation, stress, infections and anesthesia/surgery.
- Be prepared for unplanned hospitalizations, as the percentages predict that they will happen sooner or later with Parkinson's disease.

Neurologist Care and Reduction of Hospitalizations

Allison Willis at the National Parkinson Foundation Center of Excellence and her colleagues at the University of Pennsylvania addressed the impact neurologist care had on hospitalization.[49,50] Willis reported that the involvement of a neurologist in the care of Parkinson's disease patients reduced morbidity, decreased nursing home placement and improved overall survival. She examined Medicare beneficiaries over a four-year period and identified those with a diagnosis of Parkinson's disease. There were 24,929 cases, and of those cases, 13,489 had a neurologist involved in their outpatient care. Hospitalizations and repeat hospitalizations occurred less in those who had seen an outpatient neurologist. Those with an outpatient neurologist were less likely to be hospitalized for psychosis, urinary tract infection or traumatic injuries.

The bottom line for the Parkinson's disease patient is that having a neurologist involved in your care makes a big difference. Morbidity, mortality and hospitalization are all curbed by the involvement of a specialist. This current study did not assess whether a neurologist was actually involved in a patient's care when checked in to the hospital but did assess whether the patient had seen a neurologist as an outpatient prior to their hospitalization. The main finding of the study was that neurologist care reduced hospitalization risk. Outcomes would likely be even better if Parkinson's patients could have regularly scheduled visits with a neurologist. The dream scenario would be for patients to retain a neurologist with Parkinson's disease specialty training, though worldwide there are few of these available.51

Take Home Points:

- Previously in "Parkinson's Treatment: 10 Secrets to a Happier Life," we emphasized how to survive a hospitalization.6 A better plan is to try to avoid the hospitalization.
- Following up regularly with a neurologist is helpful (a few times a year), and if possible, a movement disorders-trained neurologist is optimal.
- When a management issue emerges in the care of a Parkinson's disease patient, be aggressive and try to schedule an urgent visit with your neurologist.
- If there is an emergent balance issue and any risk of falling, try not to walk unassisted. If possible, do not leave a Parkinson's disease patient in this condition alone. Guard against falling until the doctor and physical therapist can optimize medications, administer physiotherapy and prescribe assistive devices and techniques to avoid falling. Falling will eventually result in broken bones, hospitalizations, and in some cases, nursing home placement.
- Hallucinations and paranoia should be treated with medication optimization and in some cases Quetiapine (Seroquel) and Clozaril (clozapine) but not typical dopamine blockers (e.g. Haldol). Pimavanserin may be a useful alternative when available.

- Medicines such as dopamine agonists, amantadine, MAO-B inhibitors and drugs to reduce frequency of urination can all potentially lead to confusion, hallucinations or disorientation. Though Sinemet (Madopar or Parcopa) can also contribute, when simplifying regimens, many experts will temporarily simplify to Sinemet-only regimens when a patient is in the hospital and suffering from confusion.
- Metoclopramide (Reglan) is frequently given to Parkinson's disease patients after elective procedures to improve gastrointestinal mobility. This drug will worsen Parkinson's disease.
- Compazine and Phenergan are anti-nausea and headache drugs frequently given by primary care doctors and will worsen Parkinson's disease symptoms.
- Antibiotics may affect the absorption of Parkinson's disease medications and result in a worsening of symptoms.
- A great caregiver who can function as an aggressive advocate will provide the best opportunity for a Parkinson's disease patient to avoid a hospitalization.
- There is a one in three risk for hospitalization (ER or inpatient) each year in Parkinson's disease, but after being hospitalized the risk jumps to one in two.

·→⇒ ⇐←·

Chapter 7

Advancing Deep Brain Stimulation Technology, Earlier Intervention and Dopamine Pumps

"I'd say we're all just ghosts on a wire seeking the prick of an electric thought."

-Robert Fanney

ALIM-LOUIS BENABID, AN accomplished doctor, was not known beyond his specialized field. He was a professor of neurosurgery at the Joseph Fourier University in Grenoble, France from 1978 to 2007. His routine duties included treating people debilitated by the symptoms of Parkinson's disease by placing small lesions into deep regions within their brains. One day, Benabid had a "what if" moment that would forever alter the treatment of Parkinson's disease. More importantly, it would radically and positively impact the lives of many people.

On the operating room table was an elderly man who was afflicted by pain and tremors. Benabid utilized a technique referred to as intraoperative mapping, and as a routine he gathered a detailed physiological brain map. Benabid would obsessively check and double check his map to confirm localization of the "sweet spot." He was aware from his thousands of hours of intraoperative experience that the sweet spot was the precise location within the brain that if tickled would result in relief of Parkinson's symptoms. He also knew that if he missed the spot, there would be no relief, and in some cases it could precipitate severe side effects.

Benabid passed a large test probe several centimeters below the brain's surface. Initially, the results were as he predicted; the tremor worsened when he stimulated through the probe with a series of very slow pulses. In contrast, it improved when he stimulated with faster pulses. What happened next was the real breakthrough. Instead of burning a hole in the brain, Benabid decided to change course. It would be hard to not to overstate the significance of this moment because of the tens of thousands of Parkinson's disease and tremor patients whose lives would be forever transformed by that decision. Instead of heating the tip of the test probe and placing a tiny lesion deep inside the brain, he withdrew it and placed what would later be referred to as a deep brain stimulation (DBS) lead.144-148

Previous to Benabid's use of a chronically-implanted DBS lead to treat the symptoms of Parkinson's disease, conventional treatment was to make a brain lesion to "disrupt the disruption" in a rogue brain circuit that was stuck in a state of abnormal oscillation.

One of the amazing observations about the human brain is that its normal functions seem to be dictated by rhythmic oscillations that continuously repeat over and over, much like a popular song on the radio. The oscillations change and modulate, and they act to control various human behaviors. If an oscillation "goes bad," it can result in a disabling tremor or alternatively in many of the other symptoms of Parkinson's disease.

That day in the operating room, Benabid decided to remove the lesion probe he had used hundreds of times before and replace it with a wire that had four metal contacts at the tip. This wire, later referred to as a DBS lead, was connected to an external battery source. Benabid and his neurology colleagues could program the device using a small, old-fashioned box with several small buttons and archaic looking switches. As simple as the system appeared, it turned out to be very powerful, allowing Benabid to individualize the settings to a possible 12,000 plus combinations. Unlike lesion therapy, this new approach provided Benabid and his team a tailored or personalized medical solution to many of the disabling symptoms of Parkinson's disease and of tremor.148

There was another potential long-term benefit to Benabid's approach. Patients holding out for stem cells, gene therapy or even a cure would remain eligible for future operations, since DBS as a therapy was completely reversible. The whole system could be extracted in a small operation that could be performed in a few short minutes. Because of the robust and undeniable benefits of this operation, it would be rare over the next two decades to hear of a patient who would request removal of their DBS device.

Deep Brain Stimulation: The Technology Expands Beyond the Original Vision

As technology has advanced, the term deep brain stimulation has turned out to be less than precise, as the idea of electrical stimulation has led to the development of an entire field sometimes referred to as "neuromodulation." The reason the term DBS is imprecise is because DBS is not always deep, not always applied in the brain and doesn't always result in stimulation of the target region.

DBS is not limited to the brain as it is now possible to excite and inhibit nerves, nerve coverings and even the spinal cord. Most people automatically think that the mechanism of action for DBS is stimulation, especially given its name. However, it turns out to be a much more complex and interesting story. Many debates and much research have been generated concerning the potential mechanisms underpinning this technology. Since the effects on humans are so dramatic, it will be critical to understand and unlock how this therapy actually works. Unlocking the secrets of DBS will likely guide the design of more rational drug therapy, gene therapy and other novel interventions.149

The first major debate about DBS occurred between two research groups living an ocean apart. The French group that discovered DBS argued that the mechanism of action was blocking or jamming of the brain's electrical activity. The argument they proposed was that DBS acted in an inhibitory way toward cells and cell-to-cell connections. Other prominent groups around the world, including Warren Grill at Case Western Reserve University and Cameron McIntyre at the Cleveland Clinic, responded to these early theories by constructing laboratory-based models to explain how the electrical current actually interacted with the neurons (brain cells) and with their billions of interconnections, which are referred to as synapses. To virtually everyone's astonishment, it was uncovered that DBS inhibited neurons and excited axons, the pipes extending out from each brain cell. This mind-blowing revelation meant that the mechanism of action for DBS was neither stimulation nor excitation. It was not simply jamming of a brain circuit. DBS was actually affecting a very large network of neural structures up and downstream from a tiny local area of electrical stimulation. This area of delivered electricity, though measuring only a meager three millimeters in diameter, proved to have dramatic effects over the entire brain and body.149-153

The early theories of how DBS worked focused on brain cells (neurons) and ignored the supporting cells known as glia and astrocytes. Those supporting cells provide critical infrastructure to facilitate all of the brain's many important functions. As an example of how critical these supporting cells can be, each astrocyte touches as many as two million synapses, which is the term used to describe the brain's interconnections. Synapses facilitate communication and direct information transfer. Forgetting about the supporting cells would be like trying to win a baseball game with only three players on your team. Electricity can act directly on neurons, astrocytes and synapses, which in turn can propagate a dumping of calcium and subsequently other important brain chemicals such as adenosine and glutamate. The chemicals that get "dumped" in response to electrical modulation are called neurotransmitters. The dumping of these neurotransmitters has emerged as an important element in facilitating the mechanism of action for DBS. It is amazing to think that DBS acts chemically as well as electrically.148,149

Since DBS likely works in many ways (electrical, chemical, excitation and/or jamming inhibition), we now believe that the electrical current sets off a complex symphony of coordinated information transfers between many brain elements and regions. This complex information transfer ultimately leads to improvement in Parkinson's disease symptoms. Since so many regions are involved in this coordinated response, we refer to this as a neural network.148,149 Phil Starr, a neurosurgeon at the University of California, San Francisco, has shown that there is a complex relationship between the cells stimulated deep in the brain and the cerebral cortex, which is the top portion of the brain. When the DBS device is turned on, the cells in the two regions fire in a new synchrony, and some of the brain's oscillations actually desynchronize.154

DBS also stimulates neurogenesis, or the formation of new brain cells. Stimulating the growth of new brain cells has opened up the hope that this technology may unlock better treatments for neurodegenerative diseases such as Parkinson's disease, Alzheimer's disease and progressive supranuclear palsy. Dennis Steindler and colleagues at the University of Florida recently showed that there are neural stem cells in the brains of Parkinson's disease patients, and they can even grow these cells off of discarded DBS leads that were removed because of device fractures. The cells seem to be drawn to and stick on the DBS lead.155-157

For some of you, DBS may seem like something out of a sci-fi movie, but with all the medical and technological advances that have been recently accomplished, what may seem futuristic has become our new reality. This means that doctors and patients have more treatment options available, and for some who suffer with tremor and other symptoms of Parkinson's disease, these alternatives can be life changing. New discoveries like DBS that lead to an improvement in disease features have the potential to unlock more of the mystery of Parkinson's disease and help many patients achieve happier and more meaningful lives.

On Whom to Operate

When we arrived at the University of Florida to build a Parkinson's disease and movement disorders center, there was no basic infrastructure in place for Parkinson's disease care. Dr. Kelly Foote (our neurosurgeon) and I were two "young guns" fresh out of fellowship training. The existing senior faculty made it clear that though they liked us, they were concerned about the potential for trouble, especially with the introduction of a potentially risky neurosurgical procedure. The message to us was: "We like you guys, but don't embarrass us." It was an understandable sentiment, as all seasoned medical school professors over the course of a career will inevitably observe dozens of purported miracle treatments. These types of treatments are usually introduced with glitz and flare, but in the majority of cases, they will completely flop. The most concerning issue to our faculty was that we were drilling holes in the skull and poking precious brain tissue. This was much riskier than a simple pill therapy. Their concerns were both understandable and also forgivable.

Over the last 10 years at the University of Florida, DBS therapy has transitioned from a crazy notion to a cool procedure and finally to a completely acceptable form of therapy. Every medical student is now required to observe one DBS operation during the course of training. Thanks to Benabid's intraoperative decision and "what if" moment, the world is moving into a bionic age.

A formidable and somewhat unexpected obstacle emerged when we set up the DBS program at our institution. We were faced with an immediate influx of 200 referrals for the procedure. Unfortunately, only eight of these referrals (four percent) were reasonable surgical candidates. Even more concerning, we observed a few dozen neurosurgeons and hospitals launch ill-fated programs. The field would learn a humbling lesson about the critical importance of choosing the right candidates for DBS. Patient selection would turn out to be the most important factor predicting the success or failure of this relatively new surgical approach. Patients who were inappropriately selected for the surgery often had disappointing and tragic results. Thus, the development of a solid DBS surgical program would require educating primary care and neurology doctors in proper screening and selection techniques, and this effort has been ongoing over the last decade. Also, most neurosurgeons and hospitals would have to inevitably reach the realization that once a Parkinson's patient is implanted, they would likely be bionic for life and would require continuing expert care. Most hospitals were not prepared to organize and invest in this type of interdisciplinary effort. Over the last decade, DBS programs appeared and offered hope to many local and regional patients. However, the majority of these programs quickly faded and ultimately dissolved.

Ironically, DBS drove a worldwide movement toward better interdisciplinary care for the Parkinson's disease patient. Prior to DBS, most care was delivered in isolation by physicians, nurses, nurse practitioners or physician assistants. The complexities of screening a DBS candidate would, in contrast to typical care, require a multidisciplinary approach. A neurologist, neurosurgeon, psychologist, radiologist and psychiatrist would all participate in a comprehensive evaluation. Over time, physical therapists, occupational therapists, speech therapists and social workers would, as a result of this process, transform into important members of this team. Together the team would make critical surgical decisions, and individually each team member would become an expert in his or her field.

Ultimately, so many people participated in the care of a single DBS patient that the process gradually shifted from multidisciplinary to interdisciplinary. Interdisciplinary care is the highest level of a patient-centric experience, and it has been utilized for decades by cancer centers and rehabilitation hospitals. Interdisciplinary care involves specialists sitting together and discussing an individual patient, which stands in contrast to consultative or multidisciplinary care, where practitioners communicate by sending notes or letters to each other. For Parkinson's disease, the birth of the interdisciplinary DBS evaluation greatly enhanced the level of care and has forged dramatic improvements in patient and family satisfaction. DBS, a surgical not medical procedure, would transform and improve the care for all Parkinson's disease patients, even those not receiving an operation.158,159

Brain Mapping

Deep within the research hallways at Johns Hopkins University, Mahlon DeLong studied a group of circuits referred to as the basal ganglia. His other colleagues and contemporaries in the lab would snatch up the more desirable and easier to decode brain regions. The soft-spoken DeLong would for many years meticulously record and sort single brain cells from Parkinson's disease basal ganglia, first in monkeys, then in humans. Slowly a coherent picture would begin to emerge, and this picture included important changes in the rate and pattern of brain cell activity.145,148 DeLong passed his craft to Jerrold Vitek, Philip Starr, Thomas Wichmann, Kelly Foote and many others including myself. We would all spend our careers refining and applying these lessons to the human DBS experience.

The procedure is a marvel of modern medicine. It requires only a dime-sized hole in the skull. The operation is performed in virtual reality on a computer screen and within minutes can be translated into a human patient. The surgeon can navigate around blood vessels and refine a region of interest to reach within a few millimeters of an intended target. A few millimeters may be small on a ruler, but it is very large in brain space. A few millimeters of brain space can be compared to the distance between Florida and California.

A famous neurosurgeon from Toronto named Andres Lozano once declared that mapping a Parkinson's disease patient's brain was similar to driving a car through Europe. As the recording microelectrode was advanced one millimeter at a time, the sound of the brain cells changed while moving from one brain region to another. He compared this change to the language changes that can be appreciated when crossing the border from one European country to another. He noted that these changes were instrumental in the process of brain mapping.

After threading several microelectrodes into a Parkinson's disease patient's brain, one can develop a three-dimensional map. This map includes both the desired target location and also the position of surrounding brain structures. There are many brain targets that can be chosen for a patient. The choice of target is usually tailored during a detailed discussion, which involves the patient and his or her DBS team. The complete map is a critical part of the DBS procedure itself because if the final DBS lead is misplaced by even a few millimeters, it can be the difference between dramatic success and miserable failure. Failure could mean a lack of benefit, but it could also mean that a patient is left with permanent stroke-like symptoms.

Once the final location for the DBS lead has been determined, it can be locked into place by a capping device. A connector wire can be attached and tunneled underneath the skin. In one final step, a battery, referred to as a neuro-stimulator, can be placed under the collarbone in an identical location. The neurostimulator is like a cardiac pacemaker. Once placed, a neurologist or nurse programmer can cycle through thousands of possible DBS programming parameters in order to optimize the settings for a patient. Optimization of the settings usually takes a few weeks to a few months and can lead to exquisite control of the many disabling symptoms of Parkinson's disease such as tremor, stiffness, slowness, and in some cases, even walking.159

Professors Benabid and DeLong together in 2014 received the Lasker Award for their research into the brain circuits underlying Parkinson's disease and for their development of DBS.148 Over thirty percent of Lasker Award winners will one day take home the Nobel Prize.

The Dream of Living Pill Free

Most people with Parkinson's disease are fed up with all the medications. In some cases, patients may have to take multiple pills every two to three hours around the clock. The price for missing a dose could be tremor, stiffness, slowness or even falling. In a cruel twist of fate, as Parkinson's disease progresses, the pills may result in uncontrollable dance-like and flailing movements. These movements have been referred to as dyskinesia, and they occur as a result of disease progression and also as a direct result of long-term use of many of the common Parkinson's disease drugs.

When a Parkinson's disease patient takes a dopamine pill, a miraculous transformation ensues. Tremor, stiffness, slowness and many other symptoms melt away within 20 to 30 minutes. A Parkinson's disease sufferer will commonly refer to the period when a pill kicks in as being "on." Conversely, when a dosage drops below a therapeutic blood level and symptoms return, they will refer to this scenario as being "off."

Many Parkinson's disease sufferers will initially respond to the medication, but inevitably and many years later develop medication-related on-off fluctuations and dyskinesia. Modern DBS has emerged as the most powerful therapy to address these types of disease related fluctuations. DBS can restore meaningful life in a large number of Parkinson's disease patients.

As the DBS story unfolded in the 1990s, many centers in Europe reported that a patient could completely stop Parkinson's medication. A transoceanic debate ensued with many North American centers advocating a less aggressive approach to medication reduction. Two decades later, the entire field now appreciates that it is very rare to terminate all Parkinson's medications following a DBS operation. We have learned that medication reduction occurs in some but not all patients, and that it is more common when two DBS leads are employed (one on each side of the brain) into a very specific brain region called the subthalamic nucleus. In some cases, apathy, walking problems and other issues will emerge if Parkinson's medications are stopped or reduced too quickly. Thus, the hope of offering Parkinson's disease sufferers pill-free existences remains largely elusive. Neuromodulation has, however, emerged as a powerful complement to pharmaceutical options and as a means to better manage one's life.

Advancing Technology

One remarkable fact about DBS therapy is that the hardware has changed very little since Benabid's experiment. The brain lead, the connector wires and the battery technologies have only been slightly improved. The FDA currently has approved only one DBS device for Parkinson's disease patients, and it is well known that better technologies are languishing as they snake their way through the trenches of a difficult FDA approval process. The techniques for delivering currents and securing the electrodes remain fundamentally unchanged. Despite the lack of a new DBS technology, penetration of the device into communities all over the world has been explosive, with nearly 100,000 Parkinson's and movement disorders patients having been transformed into bionic existences.

Why haven't more DBS devices become available over the past two plus decades? The answer to this question is complex. Studies validating the current DBS technology for Parkinson's disease have revealed clinical outcomes that were more robust than anyone expected. When I entered the field in the mid-to-late 1990s, the top experts advised me against pursuing DBS research, as they were sure the therapy would disappear and be replaced by better medicines. Not only has the therapy survived, but the clinical and financial success of DBS has snowballed, and the effect has drawn more patients, more researchers and more venture capitalists into the device arena. While many pharmaceutical companies have flirted with the next big Parkinson's drug, none of these efforts have been robust and most have flopped. A multi-billion dollar industry attracts all kinds of people, and the infusion of novel scientific ideas and fresh cash has brought at least a half a dozen new companies into the electric brain sphere. Each company offers an improvement or tweak to the currently available DBS system, and this is promising for the hope of advancements in the near future.

So what will it take to move the DBS field forward? A critical first step will be to develop an understanding of the needs of the Parkinson's disease sufferers. Patients and families currently seek treatment to address the symptoms that are not adequately addressed by medications and current DBS therapy. (For example, thinking issues and falling.) Second, the therapy will need to be safe, and clinical trials will need to be sufficiently robust and demonstrate benefit greater than the placebo effect. (For example, improvement greater than would be predicted by chance). Third, the therapy must be cost effective and incrementally better than all existing therapies. Any hope of moving the technology and ultimately the field forward will need to address these three major hurdles.

There have been important and recent research advances in DBS device development. First, there are many new DBS lead designs. Most of the new designs will enable the electrical current to be administered to more specific regions of the brain, thereby enhancing benefits and reducing side effects. Second, the type of electrical current we now utilize is referred to as a voltage-driven system. In this voltage-driven paradigm, there can be shifts over time in the actual size and shape of the electrical field that is delivered to the brain tissue. Newer stimulators, like the one designed by St. Jude Medical (Plano, Tx), will use a constant current device that will smooth tissue delivery and improve the effectiveness of the therapy. A third issue that has emerged is battery life. Clinicians and patients have a critical need for longer lasting, and in some cases, rechargeable batteries. Better battery lives will mean fewer replacement surgeries and less of a chance for battery failure and return of symptoms. These new approaches and products have already begun to appear and are working their way through the FDA approval process.

Patients have also begun to demand sleeker and smaller devices as a box protruding from the chest area is unattractive and undesirable. They would also prefer the wires and caps on the head not stick up like horns (e.g. a countersinking procedure to hide the wires). It would also be preferable to most patients to eliminate the connector wire that attaches the lead in the head to the box in the chest. Finally, it would be ideal to be able to program the device from a remote location. Imagine the day when a doctor can see you by video and tune your device without the need to change out of your pajamas or leave your house. All of these advances are coming soon.

Another encouraging development is the ability to tailor or personalize a therapy for an individual patient. We previously targeted our surgery to one specific area of the brain for all Parkinson's sufferers. With all the advancements, we are able more and more to hone in on specific bothersome symptoms. For example, one brain target may be best for tremor, while another is preferable for speech, and still a third target would be chosen for walking. Patients would choose the target based on their needs. For example, a chef may choose a target that maximally suppresses tremor, while a trial lawyer or teacher may choose a target that preserves speech. Also, we are no longer limited to one or even two brain leads. The ability to place multiple DBS leads into a single patient over time as his or her disease evolves and new symptoms emerge is quickly becoming a reality.

Combining Electricity with Other Therapies

As the mechanisms underpinning the success of the electric brain come into focus, the possibilities and potentials are exploding. Now that we understand that changes in the rate and pattern of neuronal cell firing are responsible for many of the observed benefits, we can harness this information to develop newer and better therapies. Additionally, the realization that many of the clinical benefits result from changes in brain chemicals such as adenosine and glutamate can also help in facilitating the design of more rational drug therapies.

One provocative area of research and development has been the idea to combine DBS with other novel therapies. Specifically, the idea of utilizing a DBS lead as a catheter that can inject genetic therapies, stem cells and growth factors. The general idea is to combine powerful symptomatic therapy such as brain stimulation with approaches that may have the potential to slow down disease progression. Greg Gerhardt and Craig van Horne at the University of Kentucky have been engaged in a human experiment to develop this approach. The idea of "DBS plus" will hopefully offer the best of both worlds.

An Electric Biomarker

The newest Holy Grail in science and in Parkinson's disease will be the development of a biomarker. The National Institutes of Health defines a biomarker as "a characteristic that is objectively measured and evaluated as an indicator of normal biologic processes, pathogenic processes, or pharmacologic responses to a therapeutic intervention." In layman's terms, a biomarker is an indicator that one has or does not have a disease (i.e. a blood test that may reveal the diagnosis of Parkinson's disease). When it comes to the electric brain, scientists have raised the possibility of an electrical biomarker. The general idea is that disease activity could be monitored by an electrical signal that is being naturally emitted by specific brain regions. So instead of using the biomarker to diagnose the disease, doctors would use the abnormal electrical patterns to direct treatment – in this case, electrical treatment of Parkinson's.

It has recently become possible to record the brain after DBS and capture the signals in real time. Previously, the brain could only be recorded during the actual operating room procedure. The type of signal that can now be collected is called a local field potential or LFP. A LFP is a special measurement of the brain's native electrical current and also measures its oscillatory properties or tendency to vibrate in certain patterns. In Parkinson's disease, research has revealed an important LFP called the beta band. This band changes when medication or DBS is administered. Understanding electrical biomarkers will allow the development of smarter devices. The hope is that new devices will sense a particular abnormality, such as a beta band, and automatically respond. The result is called an on-demand paradigm. In on-demand circuits, electrical abnormalities can be addressed by applying current to the brain. The idea of on-demand systems is to solve brain problems as they emerge and before the development of a particular clinical issue or symptom. Another term for on-demand has been responsive DBS. Thus the era of personalized medicine has arrived.

A Shift Back to GPi DBS

A huge question facing Parkinson's disease patients and clinicians has been: what is the best target for deep brain stimulation (DBS)? Over the years, two main brain regions have emerged as possibilities; the subthalamic nucleus (STN) and the globus pallidus internus (GPi). Though each target has had defenders, most centers have gravitated toward utilizing only STN DBS. A series of recent trials, however, will likely change this simple practice pattern into a more complex and tailored approach.

Weaver and colleagues published the long awaited three-year data that was derived from the VA-NIH STN vs. GPi DBS for Parkinson's disease trial.

Patients were randomly assigned to a GPi or a STN brain target, and though the original trial had more subjects, this long-term follow-up cohort was relatively large for a surgical trial (GPi n=89 and STN n=70). The primary outcome was "motor function on stimulation/off medication using the Unified Parkinson's Disease Rating motor subscale," and patients were followed for a total of 36 months. Motor function, as in the original trial, improved similarly in both groups. The surprise was that the Mattis Dementia Rating Scale and other neurocognitive/thinking measure scores such as the Hopkins memory test "declined faster for STN than GPi patients." Overall, quality of life was improved in both groups, though it was overall diminished from the previously reported 24-month follow-up. This worsening of quality of life was thought to be due to disease progression.160,161

The recent VA-NIH Cooperative study focusing on STN vs. GPi DBS validated previous reports by Anderson and also reports from the NIH COMPARE DBS randomized trial. All of these STN vs. GPi DBS studies have collectively demonstrated similar motor efficacy when using either brain target when applied to patients with advanced fluctuating Parkinson's disease. Though many neurologists and neurosurgeons may have prematurely rushed to adopting STN over GPi DBS, accumulating evidence has underscored a critical importance of carefully and thoughtfully studying DBS targets through the application of appropriate clinical trials.162

The results of the current study were largely forecasted by a 2005 editorial that provided an illustrated cartoon entitled "The Rematch." The editorial compared a very popular STN DBS target against the less utilized GPi. The cartoon even went so far as to place boxing gloves on each target. There was speculation that the GPi target would "make a return," and that in the future, DBS targets would be chosen on a symptom-specific basis.163,164 If we fast-forward to the present, it seems that this projected scenario is quickly becoming a reality.

The current VA study by Weaver and colleagues revealed specific advantages of the GPi DBS target. The most important reported finding was the worsening of cognitive/thinking function in the STN group. This finding has practical implications for patients. If you are considering a DBS and you have cognitive or thinking issues, you and your team should consider implantation into the GPi target. Additionally, sometimes detailed cognitive testing will uncover previously unknown but potentially important symptoms. Another important take home message is that although medication reduction occurs more commonly with the STN brain target, there seems to be more flexibility in adjusting medications if you choose the GPi target. The ability to have enhanced flexibility when making medication adjustments will likely be important as DBS patients experience natural disease progression and worsening of symptoms.161

The data from the Weaver study also revealed that in STN DBS, there was a gradual loss of the "additive effect of medication to stimulation." This point led the accompanying editorial to question whether "GPi stimulation would be more compatible with long-term medical therapy?"165 Additionally, the postoperative off-medication scores remained remarkably stable in the GPi target. It is unknown whether this finding represented a failure of stimulation washout, a micro-lesional effect or a disease-modifying benefit.

Maya Katz at the University of California, San Francisco recently published another paper suggesting a possible benefit in walking for patients randomized to GPi DBS. Katz looked at the VA data more carefully and concluded that although responsiveness to both GPi and STN DBS was overall similar, patients reporting a resting tremor at baseline had a better response to GPi DBS with respect to their walking. The majority of patients who receive DBS have experienced a resting tremor at some point during their Parkinson's disease and Dr. Jankovic and colleagues developed a classification of Parkinson's disease that has separated patients into tremor dominant or postural instability gait dominant phenotypes. Another point we learned from the Katz study was that the patients without tremor improved less with DBS than those with tremors.166

The results from these studies collectively suggest that clinicians weighing the possibility of DBS for their patients should not consider STN as the sole option. All of the recently available data, inclusive of this new study, supports the notion that the future of DBS patient and target selection will require a more tailored and symptom specific approach, and that both STN and GPi are viable options. All DBS patients should be sure that they are evaluated by an interdisciplinary team (neurologist, neurosurgeon, neuropsychologist, psychiatrist, PT, OT and speech therapist), and that the team has met and discussed the best approach (unilateral versus bilateral), the best target (STN vs. GPi) and the overall risk-benefit ratio. These types of pre-operative evaluations will facilitate the best chance to enhance the overall outcomes following DBS surgery.167

Earlier DBS?

Michael Schüpbach and colleagues in Germany and France decided to conduct a multi-center study to examine the potential benefits of "earlier deep brain stimulation."168 Two hundred and fifty patients were randomized to either medication therapy or DBS. The Parkinson's patients had motor fluctuations and/or dyskinesia for no more than three years. Deep brain stimulation was superior to medical therapy in this group of relatively younger (about 50 years old at Parkinson's disease onset) patients with Parkinson's disease. Another study at Vanderbilt University has been examining the application of DBS in patients prior to the onset of motor fluctuations and/or dyskinesia. This preliminary study has revealed reasonable safety, but the study was too small to determine if it was advisable for all early patients.169 Patients should not interpret these studies to mean that everyone with Parkinson's disease should receive DBS before or at the onset of dyskinesia. A more accurate interpretation would be that younger onset patients with troublesome motor fluctuations and/or dyskinesia should consider earlier DBS therapy. DBS is a powerful symptomatic therapy, but it is still brain surgery, therefore decisions to pursue surgery should be carefully considered.

New Leads and Technologies

One surprising fact about DBS technology is that the human DBS leads and the four shiny and tiny contacts contained on them have not changed much for the last two decades. One reason for the durability of DBS lead design has been the long-term beneficial effects of utilizing this simple approach. There are, however, compelling reasons to introduce new DBS lead designs into clinical practice. Each target in the brain is a different size, therefore the volume of electricity pumped into that target should be tailored to the appropriate region. Additionally, there are structures and connecting pipes (fibers) that will require selective activation to achieve the most optimal response. Finally, placing DBS leads accurately is not as easy as the general public may believe, and the ability to steer the electrical current may enhance benefits and reduce stimulation-induced side effects.

Several companies have introduced different versions of DBS leads capable of steering and shaping the current. Boston Scientific (8-contact lead, Vercise™ implantable pulse generator, Natick, MA) has a new lead in clinical trials that is capable of simultaneously activating multiple contacts and allowing the physician or expert programmer to choose the percent of electrical current delivered at each contact on the DBS lead. This DBS lead design was recently tested by Lars Timmermann and his colleagues in Germany.170 Additionally, there are twice as many contact points to stimulate on the new lead design: eight as opposed to the standard four. Eight contacts and the ability to turn on one, a few or all of the contacts (multiple source) and shape the size of the current at each contact point offers the possibility of an enhanced benefit-to-side-effect ratio. These potential benefits will need to be demonstrated in formal studies. The downside of this approach is that it may complicate the picture for a general neurologist who must program the device in a community setting. Also, the battery life of the device may be quickly depleted by using multiple sources of electrical current. The company has attempted to answer these issues by providing a user-friendly programming platform and by making the device rechargeable. The system is now part of an ongoing clinical trial.

Aleva Nanotherapeutics has a similar current-steering but novel lead design. Dr. Claudio Pollo in Bern, Switzerland, tested this new DBS lead design. Pollo and his colleagues examined shaping the DBS current by sending it in three different directions in the brain and comparing these new shapes of stimulation to standard paradigms used in commercially available devices.171 In the original Aleva study, every patient except one showed a superior benefit favoring the newer lead with directional steering of the electrical current. These researchers also reported the therapeutic benefit could be achieved by using less than half of the energy, thereby reducing battery drain. This lead is being developed as a stand-alone product that could one day be hitched to different battery sources.

A third company also recently introduced a new DBS lead design: Sapiens SBS, now owned by Medtronic, Minneapolis, Minn.172-174 The new Dutch DBS lead is unique and has 40 small circles (the active DBS contacts) spread over a large span of the DBS lead. When I first saw the technology about five years ago I dubbed it "the leopard." The reason I called it the leopard is that the lead had a lot of spots, and you could change, activate and deactivate the spots to customize, shape and steer the DBS current. The company has been working on an easy-to-use interface to customize and deliver the stimulation. The lead has been successfully tested in monkeys by Jerry Vitek at the University of Minnesota and in humans by Hubert Martens and a team of doctors from Germany.

This year we took another step forward in understanding the mechanisms underpinning the benefits of DBS. Phil Starr and his colleagues at the University of California, San Francisco implanted DBS leads on top of the brain (cortex) and also deep into the brain in a structure called the subthalamic nucleus (the most commonly chosen target for deep brain stimulation). Starr and his team found that in the motor cortex region (close to the surface of the brain) the cells were excessively synchronized to the brain's native harmony, which has been referred to by scientists as the brain's natural oscillation. When Cora de Hemptinne of Starr's team turned on the deep brain stimulator, the brain's harmony became less synchronized. Simultaneously, she was able to show that this corresponded to the motor features of Parkinson's disease improving.154 This change in the brain's network likely underpins much of the benefit we see from applying electricity to the human brain.

We are now realizing a DBS device can possibly be "on" or activated only when needed. Our group recently experimented with this possibility in a NIH study we performed with a graduate student, Nick Maling, who went on to Case Western University in Cleveland, Ohio and Justin Sanchez, who now directs the 80 million dollar DBS subnets project for the United States government (DARPA). When Maling and Sanchez were with us, we became interested in the idea that in Tourette syndrome patients could administer DBS on a limited duty cycle (i.e. the device would not be on all the time) and that we could possibly use this to control tics. In our original patients we demonstrated the proof of concept that we could capture tics by administering less than two hours of stimulation per day.175,176 In our latest set of experiments, Ayse Gunduz, a biomedical engineer at UF, and her student Jonathan Shute have been working on a closed-loop smart DBS system for tics and also a system to address freezing of gait in Parkinson's disease.

What Gunduz quickly realized was that real-time physiological monitoring of the brain's signals could facilitate an opportunity to "close the loop." When we say "close the loop," we are referring to a process where we perform real-time monitoring of brain waves, and we program the device to automatically respond to specific brain signals. Closed-loop stimulation is what I call "smart stimulation." We associate an abnormal brain wave with an unwanted symptom such as freezing of gait in Parkinson's disease. When the device detects the abnormal brain wave, it deploys a volley of electricity to neutralize it.177 We have experimented using technology from Medtronic (PC+S) and NeuroPace to accomplish smart stimulation. Closed-loop smart stimulation will likely be employed in clinical practice in the next five to 10 years and is already in use for the treatment of epilepsy.

There is also another intriguing possibility for improving DBS outcomes. We have been experimenting with reprogramming the software contained on the DBS battery manufactured by Medtronic (the PC) and by delivering different shaped pulses to the brain. In our preliminary study, which was performed by Umer Akbar, M.D., before he departed for Brown University in Providence,

Rhode Island to start his own movement disorders program, he was able to demonstrate that several novel pulse sequences could be as good and possibly even better for controlling the symptoms of tremor or Parkinson's disease. Warren Grill at Duke, Peter Brown at Oxford and several other colleagues have been exploring similar approaches, and it is likely we will soon use different and more novel stimulation settings for patients. Brown has also shown proof of concept for a smart DBS system in Parkinson's disease. The beauty of this approach is that we can potentially re-program the battery just like we would update an app on a cellular phone. This type of innovation will not require repeat DBS surgery.178

A Dopamine Pump

One of the common dreams shared by Parkinson's disease patients around the globe is the possibility of living a pill-free existence. One cannot blame the Parkinson's disease patient or caregiver for dreaming big. A single day walking in Parkinson's disease shoes is likely to reveal the need for dozens of pills administered day and night. In many cases, pills are taken as frequently as every hour or two. If you ask a Parkinson's disease patient to place an entire pill regimen for the day into the palms of their hands, there is a better than average chance he or she will not be able to hold all of them. Previously, there was a hope that DBS may have offered the highly sought after "pill-free existence." However, over two decades into its history it is clear that in the majority of cases, medications will still be required. There is, however, another treatment strategy on the horizon, a strategy that offers the possibility of constant stimulation of the brain's dopamine receptors through the use of a continuous dopamine infusion pump technology. Recently the first randomized controlled trial of a continuous pump infusion technology for Parkinson's disease has been published.

The trial utilized an intrajejunal (i.e. a tube inserted in the small intestine) levodopa-carbidopa intestinal gel pump infusion strategy. It was designed to collect safety and effectiveness data.179,180 The study was carefully conducted and double blind (neither the patients nor the raters knew what was administered), and the participants were randomly divided into different groups. The study was conducted in 26 centers including Germany, New Zealand and the U.S. Participants were randomized (1:1) to "immediate-release oral levodopa-carbidopa pills plus a placebo intestinal gel infusion or to levodopa-carbidopa intestinal gel infusion plus oral placebo pills." It is important to remember that everyone in the study received a pump, but half of the patients did not receive active therapy (through the continuous pump infusion). The authors were most interested in improving the amount of time spent in the "off state" following four months of therapy. Off-time improved by four hours in the pump group versus 2.1 hours in the pill group. The amount of "on" time without troublesome dyskinesia was better in the pump group when compared to the pill group (4.1 vs. 2.2 hours).

The pump is approved and available in 43 countries. The United States has lagged behind the world in adopting this new approach to Parkinson's disease therapy. However, in defense of the U.S. and the FDA, prior to the publication of the current pump trial, all previous results were based on uncontrolled evidence. The benefits of the pump have been clearly demonstrated. In this population of fluctuating patients, the data would suggest that the pump out performs standard medical therapy. The study did not enroll patients with severe dyskinesia, and it is unclear how the continuous infusion pump will perform in more severe and more disabled Parkinson's disease patients.

One of the major drawbacks to the pump approach is the need for a percutaneous gastrojejunostomy (a small feeding tube). These types of tubes can serve as nidus points for infections and other complications, and in the current study, device complications were present in 89 percent of subjects. The complications were addressable in most cases and were reported as lower than in previous pump trials.

Patients should be aware that the current version of the pump requires wearing an external device, and it also requires changing a dopamine cassette once or twice a day. The dopamine cassettes are a little smaller than a cellular phone and usually last about 14 to 16 hours. Some patients will require two cassettes, and some will need additional medications during the bedtime hours. The pumps require continuous maintenance and programming by a qualified professional. The tube connected to the stomach also requires constant monitoring for infection.

Since the continuous infusion approach received FDA approval in 2015 (Duopa, AbbVie, Chicago IL), an important step will be to compare its effectiveness to that of DBS. Patient selection for pumps versus DBS will be an immediate and critical unmet need. One question will be whether the pump technology can help debilitated patients with and without cognitive dysfunction, and can the pump help people who may be excluded from DBS therapy?

Patients should be aware that pumps are powerful symptomatic therapies but not cures; in most cases the continuous infusion pump will not address the Parkinson's disease dopamine-resistant symptoms of walking, talking and thinking. Pumps have not been shown to delay disease progression. The good news for the Parkinson's disease community is that for a subset of patients, a "pill-free existence" may be on the horizon.181

Ultrasound

Conventional DBS therapy involves drilling a dime sized hole in the skull and inserting recording as well as permanent leads directly into a brain target or region. A similar procedure is used for mapping the brain before placing a destructive lesion (thalamotomy, subthalamotomy and pallidotomy). A recent alternative ultrasound based approach has been gaining popularity. High intensity ultrasound was introduced in the 1940's and 1950's as a treatment for a variety of brain disorders. Its recent rebirth has generated a lot of enthusiasm and excitement. The repackaging of this approach has included combining ultrasound with high field MRI scanning.

Ultrasound therapy for essential tremor and potentially for Parkinson's disease has great appeal to patients and families. It does not require a scalp incision or a hole in the skull. Additionally, the therapy has advantages over gamma knife and other radiosurgical techniques. In radiosurgery the surgeon aims X-ray beams at the brain and destroys tissue. In ultrasound the tissue is still destroyed, however there is an option to apply a test-lesion prior to placing a permanent one. Radiation therapy has another disadvantage when compared to ultrasound because the X-rays can lead to necrosis (dying), and uncontrolled growth of radiation induced brain lesions. These lesions can in some cases expand uncontrollably in size, lead to delayed complications, and in one case resulted in a death.

A few important points for all patients to be aware of when considering ultrasound therapy for Parkinson's disease:

- Ultrasound is not FDA approved as a therapy for Parkinson's disease.
- The risks of ultrasound are similar to the risks of placing a conventional brain lesion (thalamotomy, subthalamotomy and pallidotomy).
- Since a destructive brain lesion can be created with both ultrasound and with conventional thalamotomy, patients should be careful to not be deceived by the ultrasound marketing (particularly videos that have gone viral), which often uses the word "scalpel-less."
- A bilateral or two two-sided ultrasound brain surgery (operating both the right and left brain) is discouraged because of a high potential for side effects (cognition, swallowing, speech). This limitation can be a serious issue and a risk for Parkinson's disease patients who may require two-sided surgery because they suffer from symptoms on both sides of their body.
- A recent study by Jeff Elias and colleagues at the University of Virginia revealed that 4/15 subjects (26.7%) had persistent sensory side effects following ultrasound therapy for essential tremor despite the use of test-lesions. One fundamental difference between ultrasound and DBS is that in DBS, re-programming of the device may in many cases can lead to resolution of symptoms.

- Microelectrode recording and physiological mapping cannot be used to refine brain targets in ultrasound therapy.

- Precision of placement of the lesion generated by an ultrasound machine has been a big hurdle for the therapy, and this area will need refinement especially as trials are conducted in Parkinson's disease patients. Patients should be educated that the ultrasound wave is generated outside the skull, and this creates a formidable challenge for millimeter sized targets deep within the brain.

- One benefit of ultrasound therapy (similar to pallidotomy, subthalamotomy or thalamotomy) is that after the procedure there are no wires, pacemakers, or follow-up visits for programming or optimization.

Apomorphine Pump

In addition to the dopamine gel trial, several trials in Europe and the U.S. are underway to test the rapidly acting apomorphine pump prototype.77,78,182 The idea has been to administer it subcutaneously or under the skin in the same place a diabetic administers subcutaneous shots of insulin. The apomorphine infusion pump has been designed to address motor fluctuations similar to the DUOPA pump.

Take Home Points:

- DBS technologies have expanded beyond the original vision of Mahlon DeLong and Alim Benabid. DeLong and Benabid recently received the Lasker Award for their groundbreaking work in DBS.

- Interdisciplinary teams and improved approaches to troubleshooting DBS have transformed the procedure to one that is better tolerated, and outcomes across the world have been improving.

- There has been a shift back toward the GPi brain target for Parkinson's disease, and choice of brain targets should be made after careful consideration of a patient's symptoms and the risk-benefit profile. The main lesson from the clinical experience has been that the DBS brain target choice should be tailored to the patient and to the symptom profile.

- It is likely that DBS will be combined with other therapies like neuro-trophic factor delivery (DBS plus).

- The mechanisms of DBS remain unknown; however, important physio-logical research has been helping us unravel the puzzle. There will likely be electrical biomarkers uncovered that will help to guide programming and management of DBS devices. These signals will facilitate closed-loop smart devices that will activate only when a troublesome symptom surfaces.

- DBS is now being applied earlier in Parkinson's disease; however, there is no concrete evidence that the risks of DBS justify implantation before the advent of motor fluctuations. This is an area where more active re-search is needed.

- There are several new DBS lead designs and programming settings that may reduce battery consumption, decrease side effects and possibly im-prove outcomes. Trials of the new lead designs and programming set-tings are needed.

- The dopamine pump is now FDA approved and may be an option for some patients with motor fluctuations; however, patient selection and management will need to be refined. The pump may facilitate decreas-ing or discontinuing medications, particularly during daylight hours.

CHAPTER 8

Stem Cells and Stem Cell Tourism

"Stem cell research can revolutionize medicine, more than
anything since antibiotics."

-Ron Reagan

OVER THE PAST several years I have had the privilege and honor to travel to many
countries as well as many regions of the United States to lecture and visit with
scientists, families and patients. Collectively these people have a heavy investment into the future of Parkinson's disease research. The most common question
I am asked is about the potential for the use of stem cells as a therapeutic treatment for symptoms as well as a cure for this neurodegenerative disease.183-188
People are keenly interested in the potential timeline for when we will see dramatic advancements in stem cell therapy.187 There was an overwhelming disappointment surrounding the George W. Bush's administration's severe limitations
that were placed on stem cell research, but there was renewed optimism under
an Obama administration that has been more supportive of stem cell research
in Parkinson's disease.6 In fact, the Obama White House has been much more
supportive of stem cell research for all diseases inclusive of Parkinson's disease.

Sometimes I find it difficult to explain stem cells to patients and family members. One simple explanation that resonates is comparing the stem cell to child
development. Early in development, parents can influence the child to differentiate into one area of life or another and develop a skill set for success in adulthood. Stem cells are a potentially self-renewing resource that can be influenced

by scientists (like parents) to differentiate into a needed tissue.186 Previously, most research efforts were geared toward the harvesting of stem cells from discarded human embryos.185,189 This type of stem cell harvesting has drawn the most controversy, mainly from religious groups with deep-seated beliefs that obtaining the cells in this manner is unethical. Recently, however, neurogenesis has been proven to occur in the adult human brain.184,186,188,190 Neurogenesis, or the formation of new cells from existing adult human brain tissue, has been an important discovery in the last decade of stem cell research. There is a region of the brain called the subventricular zone that is known to be rich in stem cells and has been referred to as brain marrow, with the comparison to bone marrow, where blood stem cells reside.186 There are now major research efforts aimed at the development of these adult stem cells that have now also been identified in other regions of the brain including the hippocampus.183-188,190,191

There are, however, significant problems with stem cells as the savior therapy for Parkinson's disease. First, when you take a cell and force it to divide you must be able to turn it on and off. If you cannot control growth of the cells, then these cells have the potential to form cancers. This limitation of stem cell therapy is an area that has drawn increasing attention from researchers and funding organizations, and pairing stem cell therapy with gene therapy, for example, may help to alleviate this issue. The other major issue with stem cell therapy is that it fails to address the complexity of Parkinson's disease. Parkinson's disease was long thought to be a simple loss of dopaminergic cells in an area of the midbrain called the substantia nigra. We are now aware that there is a much greater level of complexity to this disease and that multiple motor and non-motor circuits and regions throughout the brain are affected.192,193 Additionally, Parkinson's disease itself is likely multiple diseases with similar manifestations.194 This issue of multiple regions as well as the issue of addressing multiple motor and non-motor symptoms may prove limiting for stem cells or any transplantation strategy. Therefore, an important area of research will need to be investigation into how to encourage stem cells to repopulate and repair multiple brain circuits in many brain regions.6

Returning to the child development analogy, the stem cell is like the child. He or she has the potential to grow up and become a doctor, lawyer, accountant, painter, actor or salesperson. The parent (like a scientist) can somewhat influence the general development of the child, but ultimately he or she cannot play a central role in navigating preferred roads and avoiding perilous trails. So even if the parent (like a scientist) can get the child through college and aid in the development of a successful career, it will be impossible to for the parent to continuously shift them on and off the best roads. A stem cell can, similar to a child, be differentiated into a particular career, but the idea that it can be inserted into the brain and follow all the roads and pathways without external assistance is magical thinking. It is how to control the stem cell once it is inserted into the brain that has driven scientists crazy.

Adult (not taken from a human embryo) stem cell researchers have been hampered by a general sense of political negativity about the use of any stem cell for the treatment or cure of a neurological disease. In addition, they have been handcuffed by state governments and funding agencies who are tangled in the political questions surrounding embryonic stem cell research, even though the approach of the adult stem cell researcher should be non-controversial.

The timeline for major breakthroughs in stem cell research is at best fuzzy. We have been encouraged by the thoughtfulness of the scientists involved in the research, and we remain hopeful that more breakthroughs will emerge both with time and increased support. We hope that state agencies as well as other funding agencies will become more open to the funding of stem cell related projects, whether they are embryonic or adult-focused stem cell therapies. It is important for people interested in stem cell therapies to keep in mind that the answer may not be simply stem cell monotherapy (i.e. stem cells alone). In addition to developing on/off technology and the ability to integrate into the brain's complex circuitry, scientists should continue to keep open the possibility that a combination therapy (gene therapy, DBS, medications, etc.) may provide a more comprehensive approach to a very complex problem.

Making Induced Pluripotent Stem Cells

One of the most recent and remarkable scientific developments has been the ability of scientists to manipulate skin cells and reprogram them to become pluripotent. (They gain the ability to form multiple different cell types in the body.) This ability is the result of inducing expression of several transcription factors (which encode the genetic maps in any individual). This induction results in the generation of what have been referred to as induced pluripotent stem (iPS) cells. In initial experiments, a combination of chemicals Oct4, Sox2, Klf4 and Myc were used to induce a transition of fibroblasts (i.e. parts of skin cells) into stable and self-renewing cells that very closely resemble embryonic stem cells. Subsequently, this type of reprogramming has been demonstrated in a wide range of cell types.

Several techniques have been employed to achieve reprogramming of cells from various body tissues (somatic cells). These methods include nuclear transfer, cell fusion of somatic cells with embryonic stem cells, using skin cells in culture (from a dish in the lab) and the transduction of skin cells with defined factors and chemicals. The exact molecular mechanism of this reprogramming, however, is still uncertain. It will be necessary in the future to unlock the mystery behind why this reprogramming works in order for us to understand why the process proceeds so slowly (often over a period of several weeks), and why only a small proportion of the infected skin cells achieve iPS cell status.

iPS cell possibilities precipitate the question that is on all Parkinson's disease patients' minds: would it be possible through cell reprogramming to generate tailor-made cells as neurotherapeutics? Recent studies have shown the therapeutic application for the transplantation of iPS-derived dopamine neurons (brain cells) in a rat model of Parkinson's disease. In these studies, it was shown that dopamine neurons could be functionally integrated into the adult rat model of Parkinson's disease and that this could lead to an improvement in the clinical symptoms of the disease. Similar experiments were also performed on hemophilia A mice (iPS-derived endothelial cells into liver cells), and this also resulted in disease improvement. (hemophilia is a blood disease.) Hence, iPS cell-based strategies could become very important in the future treatment of Parkinson's disease.

Even though more work will be required before the generation of clinically applicable iPS cells, drug screening and disease modeling will be two potentially immediately useable applications for this technology. Improvements in high-throughput drug screening using iPS cells may allow for reductions in cost and improvements in the safety of drug screening (identifying new drugs to treat PD). Additionally, the techniques may help us to understand the underlying pathophysiology of the disease.195-199

There will be major challenges in the clinical implementation of therapeutic preparations derived from iPS cells. It is absolutely critical that these preparations be free of undifferentiated cells that may have the potential to form tumors. Further, the efficient purification of populations of disease-relevant cell types will be a major challenge. Finally, and perhaps most importantly, the development of techniques for the precise delivery of iPS cells into patients and the functional engraftment of the cells into the appropriate and complex basal ganglia motor and non-motor circuits in Parkinson's disease will provide the most formidable challenge. In summary, iPS cells should provide excitement for the Parkinson's disease patient, but we should also realize that a lot of the foundations for success still remain to be constructed and built upon.200,201

A High-Content Drug Screening Approach

The advances in understanding the cells and genetics underlying Parkinson's disease have made high-throughput drug screening a reality. The way this technique works is surprisingly simple. A researcher identifies a particular cell, protein, gene or element of interest. A microtiter plate is then used. These plates have thousands of little divots in them called wells, and the wells can be filled with an element chosen by the Parkinson's researcher. A robot can then apply libraries of potential drugs or therapeutic agents to each well. Many of these applied drugs are already FDA approved for other uses, thus could be immediately used on patients. The researcher then looks through the wells searching for a "hit" or an indication of an anticipated positive reaction to the combination. High-throughput drug screening using modern automated systems should make the task of searching for Parkinson's disease drugs faster and more efficient.

There are problems with this approach though. First, just because a hit is identified does not mean that it will translate into a safe and effective therapy for Parkinson's disease patients. Second, to test each Parkinson's drug in clinical trials requires thousands of patients and tens of millions of dollars. Finally, each hit may have specificity to certain genetic or other forms of Parkinson's disease, and it is possible that it will not be widely applicable to everyone with Parkinson's symptoms. One major challenge for high-throughput screening will be the advent of an efficient pipeline system that will bring relevant and high-potential Parkinson's drugs to market faster.6

Current Studies of Stem Cell Therapy for Parkinson's and Parkinsonism:

- Jaslok Hospital and Research Centre in Mumbai, India has a stem cell transplant trial that is now listed on clinicaltrials.gov as suspended.
- General Hospital of Guangzhou Military Command of PLA in Guangzhou City, China has a study of a proposed 20 patients given stem cells through an IV; it has been listed as active on clinicaltrials.gov since 2011 but no results are available.
- The Ageless Regenerative Institute in Tijuana, Mexico has a listing on clinicaltrials.gov since 2011 using Adipose-Derived Stromal Cell (ASC) implantation into the vertebral artery but no results are available.
- StemGenex in La Jolla, California has a study listed on clinicaltrials. gov in 2014 where they are testing a cellular concentrate derived from an individual's own fat, known as the stromal vascular fraction (SVF).

This company has IV, intranasal and direct injection techniques and is administering stem cells for multiple diagnoses.

What do we tell patients about stem cell therapies for Parkinson's disease?

The last decade has been one filled with hope and hype for stem cell therapies in Parkinson's disease. Unfortunately, the hype has outpaced the hope. The stem cell hope has birthed a number of predatory companies and individuals offering a stem cell cure. To date, there is no evidence that stem cells have become a viable treatment for Parkinson's disease. Patients and families should NEVER pay for a research therapy that is unsubstantiated. Anyone charging for stem cell therapies should be approached with extreme caution. Additionally, the current listings on clinicaltrials.gov reveal a paucity of current studies, and it is likely that stem cells are not ready for prime time as a therapeutic in Parkinson's disease. Stem cells are, however, powerful vehicles for testing libraries of drugs that may be effective against the symptoms of Parkinson's disease.

Take Home Points:

- Stem cell therapy has been interpreted by many patients as the great hope for a Parkinson's disease cure; however, there are several limitations of this approach.
- Stem cells can be recovered from embryos, but there is also an adult stem cell that can be utilized. There are no religious or ethical issues surrounding adult stem cells.
- Scientists can turn cells from skin and other body locations into brain cells that will produce dopamine.
- The major limitation of stem cell therapy has occurred after transplantation of the cells. Scientists have not figured out how to use stem cells to reconstitute the very complex pathways damaged in Parkinson's disease.
- Stem cells have been very useful in screening for potential Parkinson's disease drugs that can be used in clinical trials.

- Stem cell tourism is a big business. Patients should never pay for stem cell therapy. The therapy should be performed only as part of a research trial, and there should be institutional and federal oversight.

CHAPTER 9

Prions and Spreading Proteins, Vaccines and Growth Factors

"Vaccines are the tugboats of preventive health."

-William Foege

PARKINSON'S DISEASE IS a neurodegenerative condition associated with deposition of a brain protein referred to as the Lewy body. This protein deposit was named for German-born neurologist Friedrich Lewy who first observed and described these clumps in 1912. Lewy was unaware at the time, but this protein was at its core made up of a substance called alpha-synuclein. The Lewy protein can clump and spread throughout the brain, and the spread of the protein parallels the progression of Parkinson's disease. Many experts believe that much of the damage in Parkinson's disease traces to the brain's failure to process and clear this collection of alpha-synuclein containing bad proteins. As Parkinson's disease unfolds, abnormal proteins spread from lower brainstem regions to higher ones or to regions that are referred to as cortical regions. In the process of spreading, the proteins disrupt many motor and non-motor brain circuits and lead to important and often visible manifestations.202,203

Some scientists, including Nobel Prize winner Stanley Prusiner, believe that the spread of Parkinson's throughout the brain mimics infective agents. Prusiner is most famous for his discovery of proteins in the brain called prions. These proteins can, in pathological states, lead to a rapidly progressive dementia referred to as mad cow or Creutzfeldt-Jakob disease. For years, no one believed Prusiner. His colleagues, friends and the National Institutes of Health all turned their backs on him, and many laughed at his notions of disease and disease spread. History however has proven Prusiner to be correct about prion proteins. Additionally, he has recently drawn attention to the notion that proteins can migrate and act like infections in the brain. This possibility provides an intriguing explanation for how Parkinson's disease spreads within the brain tissue.204,205

Is it plausible that the brain proteins that cause Parkinson's disease are really an infection-like manifestation? As it turns out, long before Prusiner began talking about his theory, many scientists interested in the field appreciated that protein processing had already been considered to underpin this idea. Interestingly, several of these scientists described a unique reaction. When healthy dopamine cells were transplanted into human Parkinson's-diseased brains, they were found to be sick with the Parkinson's proteins.206 Though it is true that the bad proteins spread throughout the brain, it is not believed that Parkinson's disease is caused by an infection. The exact reasons for the behavior of these bad proteins and also their function remain a mystery. It is important to keep in mind that it has not been proven that Parkinson's disease is infectious and there are no documented cases of person to person spread. The prion theory of Parkinson's disease was suggested because the protein spread in the brain manifested prion-like properties.

After the initial months and years of degeneration, Lewy bodies begin to creep beyond the deep brain regions and insidiously leak into areas involved in both motor (tremor, stiffness, slowness) and non-motor function (depression, anxiety, apathy, sexual dysfunction, memory, thinking). Patients suffering from neurological disorders and their families need to appreciate that in brain real estate, there is nothing more important than "location, location, location." Location dictates symptoms.207-211

A new therapy for Parkinson's disease has recently undergone and completed human safety testing. The Austrian company AFFiRiS AG launched a two-year clinical trial of a vaccine that was designed to stop Parkinson's disease progression.

The idea underpinning the Parkinson's vaccine is simple. Patients will receive four injections. The hope is that the injections will stimulate an immune system response against alpha-synuclein and antibodies will be raised and will attack bad brain proteins, ultimately clearing them. Thirty-two human Parkinson's disease patients were part of a two-year safety and tolerability study named the PD01A project. The preliminary results of the study revealed the vaccine was safe and well-tolerated, though relatively few people were tested. Half of those in the study developed antibodies against alpha-synuclein, and for those patients the investigators believed that the appearance of antibodies was a positive sign. Why some patients did not develop antibodies remains unknown, and a follow-up study will address the use of booster vaccine shots.

It is important to keep in mind that not all experts believe that removal of these brain proteins will result in clinically meaningful changes and disease modification. Additionally, we must keep in mind that one highly publicized attempt to remove amyloid plaques in Alzheimer's patients led to serious safety concerns and termination of a vaccine study known as AN1792. Several patients in the Alzheimer's study developed a serious brain inflammation called a meningoencephalitis.

What patients need to know about the vaccine is that it is still in the very early stages of testing, but the idea is novel and the approach is promising. The hope is that clearing Parkinson's-associated brain proteins will translate into disease modification. A similar approach is also being tested in other diseases such as Alzheimer's disease, diabetes and atherosclerosis.

Using a different approach, Prothena and Roche are developing monoclonal antibodies (i.e. antibodies that are specific and only bind to a single substance) that will directly target alpha-synuclein. What is the difference between monoclonal antibodies and a vaccine? The monoclonal antibodies are injected into the patient as a direct therapy, whereas the vaccine shot stimulates the immune system to produce antibodies against alpha-synuclein. Both are considered under the umbrella of "immunotherapies." Two dose-finding and human safety trials of the first Parkinson's monoclonal antibody PRX002 have been performed, and preliminary data has shown the therapy to be safe.

It is important to keep in mind that not all experts believe that removal of these brain proteins will result in clinically meaningful changes and disease modification. Additionally, we must keep in mind that one highly publicized attempt to target amyloid in Alzheimer's patients led to serious safety concerns and termination of that vaccine study (AN1792).

What patients need to know about the vaccine and monoclonal antibodies is that both are still in the very early stages of testing, but the idea of boosting immunity and using immunotherapy is novel and promising. Safety, tolerability and clinical efficacy will all need to be demonstrated before the vaccine and the monoclonal antibodies can move into the next phase of clinical testing. There are also several animal models and approaches being tested.[212,213] Our hope is that clearance of the Parkinson's-associated brain proteins will translate into disease modification.[74,213-217] A similar approach is also being tested in other diseases such as Alzheimer's disease, diabetes and atherosclerosis. The immunotherapies are definitely something to get excited about.[218]

Two current human vaccine strategies:

PD01: α-synuclein vaccination (AFFiRiS)

- Breaks down α-synuclein accumulations in the brain.
- Stimulates antibodies against the protein α-synuclein.
- Phase I safety study was positive, and we await effectiveness and efficacy studies.

PRX002: α-synuclein antibody (Prothena)

- Intravenous infusion (IV) of a monoclonal antibody directly targeting α-synuclein.
- Phase I safety study was positive, and we await effectiveness and efficacy studies.

Trophic Factors

One very exciting area of Parkinson's disease therapeutics has been the development of gene therapies and trophic factors. Trophic factors are proteins that are important to cell development. They play a critical role in promoting brain cell survival. A few years ago, glial cell-derived neurotrophic factor (GDNF) was pumped into human Parkinson's disease brains, but the therapy was not proven to have a robust clinical effect and in some cases was associated with unacceptable adverse events. Another pill called Cogane, also a neurotrophic therapy, failed in a human trial.6

CERE-120 was a trial that utilized an adeno-associated virus to deliver a protein, called neurturin, to the brain. The idea of the trial was to rescue some of the dying brain cells and improve motor function. In the first pilot trial of this approach, conducted a few years ago, neurosurgeons drilled small holes into the skulls of patients and inserted the therapy through a pipe called a guide cannula. The neurosurgeons placed the neurturin therapy directly into a brain structure called the putamen. The trial results indicated that there was no benefit at the 12 month time point for neurturin when compared to placebo injections, but there was a possible benefit when following patients out as far as 15 months. The investigators decided to repeat the trial, increase the dose of neurturin and deliver it into two brain locations: the putamen and the substantia nigra. The investigators also decided to lengthen the follow-up period to 15 months to account for possible delayed benefits that may have been missed on the pilot trial. The primary outcome, which was the improvement in Parkinson's disease motor scores (the UPDRS), was not achieved.219-221

Should the results of the CERE-120 (neuturin) and other neurotrophic factor trials be a complete disappointment to the Parkinson's disease community? I would argue no. First, this trial demonstrated the safety of using adeno-associated gene therapy in human patients, and this has now been performed several times in real Parkinson's disease patients. The ability to safely deliver trophic factors like neuturin using technologies such as gene therapy will be important for future trials with various novel therapeutic agents. Second, we learned a great deal about delivery systems and how hard it is to get any therapy across the blood-brain barrier. The blood-brain barrier is designed to protect the brain, but it has introduced significant challenges for the therapeutic development of drugs targeting Parkinson's disease symptoms. Finally, we were humbled that despite promising animal trials, human trials did not pan out.6

Virus-Based Approaches

A common question asked by Parkinson's disease patients is "What is gene therapy?" Gene therapy is placing genetic information (DNA) into the cells and tissues of humans with Parkinson's disease. In the purest form, a defective part of the genome is replaced with a new copy. The most interesting part of the evolving story of gene therapy has been the use of a virus as a vector to carry genetic information to the brain. Viruses can be deactivated and safely used for this purpose, and they can be tagged with either genetic material or neurotrophins. Neurotrophins are a family of proteins that induce survival, development and proper functioning of brain cells.

There have been three major gene therapy studies or neurotrophin trials in addition to the above described neuturin trial in humans with Parkinson's disease. The first trial aimed to deliver amino acid decarboxylase and was sponsored by a company called Avigen. A brain enzyme, amino acid decarboxylase, enhances the effectiveness of dopaminergic replacement medicines like levodopa (Sinemet or Madopar). This therapy was aimed at improving motor symptoms, reducing medication dosages and reducing side effects. In the first study, there was some mild improvement noted, but the therapy fell short of its anticipated potential. It did, however, prove to be safe.222,223

Another gene therapy approach focused on an enzyme called glutamic acid decarboxylase (GAD) and was sponsored by Neurologix. Michael Kaplitt and Matt During reported in The Lancet in 2007 the "safety and tolerability of gene therapy with an adeno-associated virus (AAV) borne GAD gene for Parkinson's disease: an open label, phase I trial."224

The subthalamic nucleus (STN) is a brain structure that spews a chemical called glutamate onto another structure in the brain called the globus pallidus. Many treatment schemes have focused on controlling or neuromodulating the output from the STN region. One such approach has been inserting a lead into the brain and introducing electricity to change the firing pattern emanating from the STN (deep brain stimulation). Kaplitt and colleagues developed an alternative and innovative approach by using gene therapy to change the STN from a chemically-excitatory nucleus to a chemically-inhibitory one.

What they proposed and pulled off was very clever. They measured the safety, tolerability and preliminary effectiveness of the "transfer of the glutamic acid decarboxylase (GAD) gene with adeno-associated virus (AAV) into the STN of patients with Parkinson's disease." The original study had only 11 patients, and the group was similar to those typically chosen to undergo deep brain stimulation (under 70 years old with on-off medication related Parkinson's fluctuations and only minimal cognitive dysfunction). The most important outcome was that there were no adverse events related to the gene therapy. Significant improvements in the motor scores of the patients were also seen, but the results were not of the magnitude that would be required to rock the field.

The amount of change in the motor scores was similar to what has been observed following deep brain stimulation, although longer term follow-up will be needed. Many experts believe that gene therapy has a high "bar" to pass, as the results of deep brain stimulation have provided excellent benefits in a similar group of patients. Preliminary analyses point to the benefit (similar to deep brain stimulation) as being predominantly in motor function and not in areas of non-motor or levodopa-resistant symptoms (depression, sleep, gait, balance, communication, etc.). No one knows if changing the excitatory function of the nucleus into an inhibitory function will affect learning, but this is a point that will require close follow-up.

The most important finding of the Kaplitt study was that gene therapy was successfully used in humans with Parkinson's disease and the success will hopefully open the door to future gene therapies as well as combination therapies (genes plus stem cells, genes plus medications or genes plus deep brain stimulation).6

Another new therapy is ProSavin (Oxford BioMedica), and Stéphane Palfi and colleagues published their approach in The Lancet in 2014. The authors examined safety and preliminary efficacy of ProSavin injection into a structure in the brain called the putamen. The virus used was a lentivirus which is slightly different than the previous trials that used adenovirus. There were three genes delivered in this therapy: aromatic amino acid dopa decarboxylase, tyrosine hydroxylase and GTP-cyclohydrolase 1. The aim of the study was to transform brain cells and change them into dopamine-secreting cells. The 15 initial patients tolerated the therapy and also showed some signs of improvement.225

The four published gene and trophic-factor therapy approaches were all clever ways to address disabling symptoms in Parkinson's disease. What will it take though for gene therapy to deliver a cure? Ultimately, we need to better understand the target and type of patient we will need to treat with this approach. We will need a target that if modified will arrest the progression of Parkinson's disease, and we will need to deliver the gene and/or trophic factor early enough in the disease to make a difference for the patient.6,226,227

Current Trials of Neurotrophic Factors

ProSavin

- Drug delivered by a virus into a part of the brain called the putamen.
- Genetic material inserted that helps enzymes that work on dopamine-tyrosine hydroxylase, AADC and cyclohydrolase 1.
- These enzymes stimulate the production of dopamine.
- This is an active trial on clinicaltrials.gov.
- Convection enhanced delivery/AAV2-GDNF
- This is an active trial recruiting on clinical trials.gov with the PI in Bethesda, Maryland at NIH.

Peripheral Nerve Grafts Implanted During DBS Surgery

- This is an active trial on clinicaltrials.gov at the University of Kentucky in Lexington where investigators implant nerve fibers into the substantia nigra at the same time they perform subthalamic deep brain stimulation.

Small Interfering RNA Approach

Small interfering ribonucleic acid (RNA), also known as siRNA, is a class of double-stranded RNA molecules that can interfere or promote expression of a particular gene. The interference technique can be used to determine the function of a particular gene and also to develop targets for drug therapy. Your body's genetic code is made up of four nucleotides (molecules that make up your DNA and RNA): adenine, guanine, cytosine and thymine. These four nucleotides are carefully ordered, and they are transcribed into something called RNA. RNA is then transcribed or read to make the body's proteins. The technology of siRNA was designed as a way to use double strands of RNA to alter the expression of your DNA.

The siRNA technique was first described in London by David Baulcombe's laboratory which was focused at the time on gene splicing in plants. Baulcombe had no idea how important this technique would become. Later, Thomas Tuschl published a paper in the journal Nature introducing the technique to mammals, and instantly with this single publication, the field acquired a promising new therapeutic tool. Today, there is great hope that this technique can be applied across many diseases. There have been recent attempts at using siRNA to treat macular degeneration, Ebola virus and other diseases. To date, however, the technology has not proven to be a robust one within human conditions, and issues have arisen such as immune responses (e.g. your body attacking itself) that can be accidentally set off by the introduction of siRNA.

Interestingly, in macular degeneration the siRNAs were designed to knock down the gene important to blood vessel growth also known as angiogenesis. Researchers found that the siRNAs were effective, not because of a direct effect against the gene, but due to the body's own immune response. Future trials will need to take this factor into consideration.6

In Ebola, preliminary findings have been more dramatic and more promising. Researchers from Boston University believe they have uncovered a technique using siRNA that may prove to be the first treatment for this devastating virus. Preliminary trials on primates have been promising, and it was approved (TKM-Ebola) for use in human Ebola in 2014. We will hopefully soon understand if this approach was effective.

Converting siRNA into a therapy for Parkinson's disease has, however, proven to be challenging. When siRNA was used to target the gene that leads to alpha-synuclein overexpression in Parkinson's disease, it did not have the expected robust and positive effects. siRNA has baffled Parkinson's disease researchers in critical areas such as the best way to deliver the therapy, what target to aim for and how to handle the unexpected and unanticipated off-target side effects. (Off target refers to unintended consequences on other cells and tissues.)

If researchers can devise better ways to harness siRNA therapy, it could prove a very powerful symptomatic treatment or even a cure for some of the genetic forms of Parkinson's disease.6

The Optogenetic Approach

Francis Crick, one of the most famous scientists of our generation, described a double helix structure that is now known to characterize human DNA. He published this discovery in 1953 with his colleague James Watson. In the 1970s, Crick discussed in Scientific American a wish list for future discoveries, including the use of light to control human cells. Light science and light therapy have since been considered both "crazy and far-fetched." However, recent discoveries in the early 21st century have dramatically changed this point of view. Thanks to some very clever scientists, a new field called optogenetics was born. In the past several years, it has developed into one of the most important areas in Parkinson's and also science.

What is optogenetics? "Opto" refers to placing light onto the brain to activate channels and/or enzymes that will ultimately change brain cell firing. The technique is specific and has the potential to add or delete firing patterns from the brain's native cells. Additionally, brain cell firing can be manipulated at precise millisecond intervals. The fiber-optic light source can be mounted on the skull or placed deep within the brain.

The "genetics" part of optogenetics utilizes a simple virus carrier system to deliver genes to the brain. The most important of these genetic deliveries has been opsin, which is one of the structures that can be turned on by the light. The most important known opsin used for this technology is Channelrhodopsin-2. This opsin was derived by scientists from algae-based systems. By shining light onto the inserted genetic alteration (opsin), scientists can probe the brain's inner conversations (firing of cells). The technique has allowed investigators to move past the classical genetic animal manipulations and models and obtain greater specificity in their experiments.

Alexxai Kravitz and colleagues from the pioneering optogenetics group at Stanford University published an important paper about Parkinson's disease in Nature Medicine. The authors were able to demonstrate that optogenetics could worsen or alternatively improve an animal model of parkinsonism. The investigators performed a simple experiment where they manipulated the well-established basal ganglia direct and indirect pathways, which are well known suspects implicated in the genesis of Parkinson's disease. The authors reported:

"Optogenetic control of direct- and indirect-pathway cells in medium spiny projection neurons, achieved through a viral expression of channelrhodopsin-2 in mice. Excitation of the indirect-pathway medium spiny neurons elicited a parkinsonian state, distinguished by increased freezing, bradykinesia and decreased locomotor initiations. Activation of direct-pathway medium spiny neurons reduced freezing and increased locomotion."228-230

Caroline Bass and colleagues from Wake Forest University described an optogenetic approach to controlling dopamine release. Since these publications, scores of work in optogenetics and Parkinson's disease have appeared.231-233

Activating brain circuits by using both light and genetics has evolved from a science-fiction dream into a reality. The technique will likely be refined over the next decade, and it will have tremendous potential to unlock important clues underlying the disease processes ultimately responsible for Parkinson's disease. Optogenetics may also open novel therapeutic possibilities. The technology will help us shine a light on this common and often disabling human neurodegenerative condition, but whether it can be harnessed or combined with stem cells or other therapies to move us toward a cure remains unknown. It is likely we will in the near future observe Channelrhodopsin-2 inserted into target-specific cell types in the Parkinson's brain, hopefully as a powerful symptomatic therapy. It is also likely that the founder of optogenetics, Karl Deisseroth, will one day receive the Nobel Prize.6,234

Take Home Points:

- Abnormal proteins in the brain called Lewy bodies can spread from one brain region to another similar to the infectious agent called a prion.
- Understanding the spread of these proteins has stimulated an important discussion as to how we may address Parkinson's disease by stopping the spread.
- Several immune modulatory or vaccine-based approaches have been introduced and are in trial.
- We do not yet know if clearing the protein from the brain will improve the symptoms of the disease or affect disease progression.
- Other promising therapies such as neurotrophic factors, gene therapy, siRNA and optogenetics are in various levels of development but have shown safety. There is some chance that these could be useful approaches in the future.
- For all of these new approaches, we need to better understand the target and the optimal type of patient (e.g. symptoms and genes). We will need a target that if modified will arrest the progression of Parkinson's disease, and we will need to deliver the gene and/or trophic factor early enough in the disease to make a difference for the patient.

⋯▷▣◁ ▷▣◁⋯

CHAPTER 10

The Drug Development Pipeline

"The United States has an active pharmaceutical industry that
has brought huge benefits to the U.S. public. Most Americans,
who benefit from these advances, have little understanding of
how difficult it is to create an important new medical therapy
and make it available to improve public health."

-Robert Jarvik

MATTHEW HERPER FROM Forbes magazine recently wrote about the drug development pipeline and the cost associated with bringing a single successful medication to the market. Eli Lilly estimated the cost to deliver a new drug as $1.3 billion dollars. Herper writes this is "a price that would buy 371 Super Bowl ads, 16 million official NFL footballs, two pro football stadiums, pay almost all NFL football players, and sell every seat in every NFL stadium for six weeks in a row." The actual cost is probably four to 15 billion dollars depending on the drug or device, and it is not unusual for the development to take more than a decade.

Luckily in Parkinson's disease, there are many drugs in the pipeline. Mort Kondracke, the famous co-host of the political show The Beltway Boys, once said that, "Practically every day, there is a story in the newspapers about a new breakthrough drug on Parkinson's." This is extremely fortunate for all of the millions of stakeholders, and especially for the patients diagnosed and for those who will be diagnosed in the future. In my last book, "Parkinson's Treatment: 10 Secrets to a Happier Life," I suggested that every patient and every family member should ask their doctor, What's new in Parkinson's disease?"6 A great follow-up question should be "What's in the pipeline doc?" In addition to those mentioned in the previous book, below is a summary of some the drugs and therapies "in the pipeline" for Parkinson's disease.

Drugs in the Pipeline:

Glutamate Receptor Antagonists and Modulators

- mGluR4 agonist dipraglurant – Targeting dyskinesia
- Amantadine extended release (ADS-5102) – Targeting dyskinesia
- Dextromethorphan/Quinidine (Nuedexta) – Targeting cognition and dyskinesia
- AFQ056 (Novartis) – Targeting dyskinesia
- SYN120 (Biotie) – 5-HT6 receptor blocker; increases acetylcholine and glutamate – Targeting cognition.
- ADX48621 (Addex) – Glutamate receptor modulator – Targeting dyskinesia.
- Amantadine/topiramate – Targeting dyskinesia, and improving fatigue.

Serotonin Agents (Targeting dyskinesia and motor fluctuations)

- Piclozotan – 5-HT1A agonist
- Eltoprazine – 5-HT1A/1B

Drugs that have been discontinued or are not currently being developed:

- Piclozotan
- Fipamezole
- Preladenant
- Famotidine
- Vipadenant
- Pardoprunox

- Aplindore
- Sumanirole
- Levodopa Methyl Ester

Different phases of the drug development pipeline recognized by the FDA (www.FDA.gov) and NIH (www.NIH.gov):

Phase I: Testing in a small group of people to evaluate safety, determine a safe dosage range, and identify side effects. Often testing is done on the general population.

Phase II: Testing in a larger group of people to examine effectiveness and verify safety. Testing is done in the disease specific population (i.e. Parkinson's disease).

Phase III: Larger scale testing of effectiveness, monitoring of side effects, comparisons to common treatments, and collection information to facilitate FDA or regulatory approval for use in humans with Parkinson's disease.

Phase IV: Testing in Parkinson's disease but also possibly other disease states. These studies examine side effects and document chronic long-term use.

Drugs in the Parkinson's pipeline must pass through phases I, II and III prior to widespread use. This process has been estimated to take on average 12 years, and to cost 350 million to 1 billion U.S. dollars.

I always share with patients and families the simple truth that our knowledge of the brain is advancing rapidly. Despite the expected failures in the majority of Parkinson's disease clinical trials, these failures will guide us to the breakthroughs.

> "Success is going from failure to failure without a loss of enthusiasm."
> - Winston Churchill

Take Home Points:

- The drug development pipeline can be confusing, and the drugs in the pipeline come and go.
- It is important to continue to monitor new drugs that may be available to you as part of clinical trials. A good method to monitor drugs that may be available as part of research studies is using the website www.clinicaltrials.gov.
- Though the cost in time and money can be tremendous for Parkinson's disease drugs, there is hope that new symptom-specific approaches will be introduced to address bothersome and previously drug-resistant symptoms (e.g. walking, talking and thinking). There is also a hope that a new future drug will meaningfully slow disease progression.

About the Author

Other Books:
Parkinson's Treatment: 10 Secrets to a Happier Life continues to be on the
Amazon.com bestseller list for two years running
http://www.amazon.com (search for Parkinson's treatment and Okun)

Michael S. Okun, M.D.
Please feel free to contact Dr. Okun with any questions or comments
Email: michaelokunmd@gmail.com
Twitter: @MichaelOkun
Website: http://parkinsonsecrets.com

Michael S. Okun, M.D. is internationally celebrated as both a neurologist
and a leading researcher. He has often been referred to as, "the voice of the
Parkinson's disease patient." He was honored at the White House in 2015 as a
Champion of Change for Parkinson's disease. He has an international following
on the National Parkinson Foundation's Ask the Doctor web-forum and he is a
Professor of Neurology at the University of Florida Health Center for Movement
Disorders and Neurorestoration. His many books and internet blog posts are
brimming with up-to date and extremely practical information.

This book is the sequel to his runaway bestseller, Parkinson's Treatment: 10 Secrets to a Happier Life, which was translated into over 20 languages. Dr. Okun is well known for infusing his readers with positivity and optimism. In his latest book he reveals the breakthroughs in Parkinson's disease that will pave the road to meaningful progress. In this book he reviews all of the recent breakthrough ideas and therapies in Parkinson's disease, and he reviews the knowledge gained which is extending far beyond a single drug or stem cell. He paints the broader and more exciting picture and reviews the portfolio of breakthroughs spanning drug, cell, vaccine, device, genetics, care, and behavior. He believes that patients and families with personal investments in Parkinson's disease should be informed and updated about all of these potential breakthrough therapies. This book informs, educates, and will inspire Parkinson's disease patients, family members, as well as health care professionals and scientists. As Dr. Okun points out, we will journey toward better treatments -- and one day a cure.

- There isn't any joking with Dr. Okun about the 10 Breakthrough Therapies for Parkinson's disease. Patients, family members, scientists, and health care providers should all read this book and prepare to become part of the exciting Parkinson's disease treatment journey. —Muhammad Ali

References

1.   Dorsey ER, Constantinescu R, Thompson JP, et al. Projected number of people with Parkinson disease in the most populous nations, 2005 through 2030. Neurology 2007;68:384-6.

2.   Kowal SL, Dall TM, Chakrabarti R, Storm MV, Jain A. The current and projected economic burden of Parkinson's disease in the United States. Movement disorders : official journal of the Movement Disorder Society 2013;28:311-8.

3.   Johnson SJ, Diener MD, Kaltenboeck A, Birnbaum HG, Siderowf AD. An economic model of Parkinson's disease: implications for slowing progression in the United States. Movement disorders : official journal of the Movement Disorder Society 2013;28:319-26.

4.   Johnson SJ, Kaltenboeck A, Diener M, et al. Costs of Parkinson's disease in a privately insured population. PharmacoEconomics 2013;31:799-806.

5.   Okun MS. The Weather Forecast for Parkinson's Disease Calls for Worldwide Economic Storm.   What's Hot in Parkinson's Disease. http://www.parkinson.org2013 March.

6.   Okun M. Parkinson's Treatment: 10 Secrets to a Happier Life: Createspace; 2013.

7.   Ascherio A, LeWitt PA, Xu K, et al. Urate as a predictor of the rate of clinical decline in Parkinson disease. Archives of neurology 2009;66:1460-8.

8.   Parkinson Study Group S-PDI, Schwarzschild MA, Ascherio A, et al. Inosine to increase serum and cerebrospinal fluid urate in Parkinson disease: a randomized clinical trial. JAMA neurology 2014;71:141-50.

9.   Schwarzschild MA, Macklin EA, Ascherio A, Parkinson Study Group S-PDI. Urate and neuroprotection trials. The Lancet Neurology 2014;13:758.

10.   Schwarzschild MA, Schwid SR, Marek K, et al. Serum urate as a predictor of clinical and radiographic progression in Parkinson disease. Archives of neurology 2008;65:716-23.

11.   Okun MS. Should I take Inosine to Raise my Uric Acid Levels and Treat my Parkinson's Disease? . What's Hot in Parkinson's Disease. http://www.parkinson.orgJanuary 2014.

12.   Simuni T, Borushko E, Avram MJ, et al. Tolerability of isradipine in early Parkinson's disease: a pilot dose escalation study. Movement disorders : official journal of the Movement Disorder Society 2010;25:2863-6.

13.   Surmeier DJ. Calcium, ageing, and neuronal vulnerability in Parkinson's disease. The Lancet Neurology 2007;6:933-8.

14.   Surmeier DJ, Guzman JN, Sanchez-Padilla J, Goldberg JA. The origins of oxidant stress in Parkinson's disease and therapeutic strategies. Antioxidants & redox signaling 2011;14:1289-301.

15.   Aviles-Olmos I, Limousin P, Lees A, Foltynie T. Parkinson's disease, insulin resistance and novel agents of neuroprotection. Brain : a journal of neurology 2013;136:374-84.

16.   Ulusoy GK, Celik T, Kayir H, Gursoy M, Isik AT, Uzbay TI. Effects of pioglitazone and retinoic acid in a rotenone model of Parkinson's disease. Brain research bulletin 2011;85:380-4.

17.   Hass CJ, Collins MA, Juncos JL. Resistance training with creatine monohydrate improves upper-body strength in patients with Parkinson disease: a randomized trial. Neurorehabilitation and neural repair 2007;21:107-15.

18.   Beal MF. Mitochondria, oxidative damage, and inflammation in Parkinson's disease. Annals of the New York Academy of Sciences 2003;991:120-31.

19.   Bloom MZ. NIH announces phase III clinical trial of creatine for Parkinson's disease. The Consultant pharmacist : the journal of the American Society of Consultant Pharmacists 2007;22:378.

20.   Writing Group for the NETiPDI, Kieburtz K, Tilley BC, et al. Effect of creatine monohydrate on clinical progression in patients with Parkinson disease: a randomized clinical trial. Jama 2015;313:584-93.

21.   Muller T, Buttner T, Gholipour AF, Kuhn W. Coenzyme Q10 supplementation provides mild symptomatic benefit in patients with Parkinson's disease. Neuroscience letters 2003;341:201-4.

22.   Parkinson Study Group QEI, Beal MF, Oakes D, et al. A randomized clinical trial of high-dosage coenzyme Q10 in early Parkinson disease: no evidence of benefit. JAMA neurology 2014;71:543-52.

23.   Shults CW, Oakes D, Kieburtz K, et al. Effects of coenzyme Q10 in early Parkinson disease: evidence of slowing of the functional decline. Archives of neurology 2002;59:1541-50.

24.   Okun MS. Halting of the Creatine Study. What's Hot in Parkinson's Disease. http://www.parkinson.org2015 May.

25.   Martin I, Kim JW, Lee BD, et al. Ribosomal protein s15 phosphorylation mediates LRRK2 neurodegeneration in Parkinson's disease. Cell 2014;157:472-85.

26.   Imam SZ, Trickler W, Kimura S, et al. Neuroprotective efficacy of a new brain-penetrating C-Abl inhibitor in a murine Parkinson's disease model. PloS one 2013;8:e65129.

27.   Foulds PG, Mitchell, J. D., Parker, A., Turner, R., Green, G., Diggle, P., Hasegawa, M., Taylor, M., Mann, D., Allsop, D. . Phosphorylated alpha-synuclein can be de- tected in blood plasma and is potentially a useful biomarker for Parkinson's disease . FASEB 2011;25:4127-37.

28.   Okun MS. Are Blood Tests for Parkinson's Disease on the Horizon? What's Hot in Parkinson's Disease. http://www.parkinson.org2012 January.

29.   Stoessl AJ, Halliday GM. DAT-SPECT diagnoses dopamine depletion, but not PD. Movement disorders : official journal of the Movement Disorder Society 2014;29:1705-6.

30.   Sadasivan S, Friedman JH. Experience with DaTscan at a tertiary referral center. Parkinsonism & related disorders 2015;21:42-5.

31.   Ofori E, Pasternak O, Planetta PJ, et al. Longitudinal changes in free-water within the substantia nigra of Parkinson's disease. Brain : a journal of neurology 2015.

32.   Okun MS. An Update on DAT Scanning for Parkinson's Disease Diagnosis. What's Hot in Parkinson's Disease. http://www.parkinson.org2014 April.

33.   Fox SH. Non-dopaminergic treatments for motor control in Parkinson's disease. Drugs 2013;73:1405-15.

34.   Pinna A. Adenosine A2A receptor antagonists in Parkinson's disease: progress in clinical trials from the newly approved istradefylline to drugs in early development and those already discontinued. CNS drugs 2014;28:455-74.

35.   Chen W, Wang H, Wei H, Gu S, Wei H. Istradefylline, an adenosine A(2)A receptor antagonist, for patients with Parkinson's Disease: a meta-analysis. Journal of the neurological sciences 2013;324:21-8.

36.   Factor S, Mark MH, Watts R, et al. A long-term study of istradefylline in subjects with fluctuating Parkinson's disease. Parkinsonism & related disorders 2010;16:423-6.

37.   Hauser RA, Hubble JP, Truong DD, Istradefylline USSG. Randomized trial of the adenosine A(2A) receptor antagonist istradefylline in advanced PD. Neurology 2003;61:297-303.

38.   Okun MS. A2A Receptor Antagonists and Parkinson's Disease Treatment. What's Hot in Parkinson's Disease. http://www.parkinson.org2013 June.

39.   Altman RD, Lang AE, Postuma RB. Caffeine in Parkinson's disease: a pilot open-label, dose-escalation study. Movement disorders : official journal of the Movement Disorder Society 2011;26:2427-31.

40.   Postuma RB, Lang AE, Munhoz RP, et al. Caffeine for treatment of Parkinson disease: a randomized controlled trial. Neurology 2012;79:651-8.

41.   Li FJ, Ji HF, Shen L. A meta-analysis of tea drinking and risk of Parkinson's disease. TheScientificWorldJournal 2012;2012:923464.

42.   Qi H, Li S. Dose-response meta-analysis on coffee, tea and caffeine consumption with risk of Parkinson's disease. Geriatrics & gerontology international 2014;14:430-9.

43.   Tan LC, Koh WP, Yuan JM, et al. Differential effects of black versus green tea on risk of Parkinson's disease in the Singapore Chinese Health Study. American journal of epidemiology 2008;167:553-60.

44.   Ellis T, Boudreau JK, DeAngelis TR, et al. Barriers to exercise in people with Parkinson disease. Physical therapy 2013;93:628-36.

45.   Shulman LM, Katzel LI, Ivey FM, et al. Randomized clinical trial of 3 types of physical exercise for patients with Parkinson disease. JAMA neurology 2013;70:183-90.

46.   Corcos DM, Robichaud JA, David FJ, et al. A two-year randomized controlled trial of progressive resistance exercise for Parkinson's disease. Movement disorders : official journal of the Movement Disorder Society 2013;28:1230-40.

47.   Ridgel AL, Vitek JL, Alberts JL. Forced, not voluntary, exercise improves motor function in Parkinson's disease patients. Neurorehabilitation and neural repair 2009;23:600-8.

48.   Okun MS. Defeating the Barriers to Implementing Exercise Regimens in Parkinson's Disease Patients. What's Hot in Parkinson's Disease. http://www.parkinson.org2013 February.

49.   Willis AW, Schootman M, Tran R, et al. Neurologist-associated reduction in PD-related hospitalizations and health care expenditures. Neurology 2012;79:1774-80.

50.   Willis AW, Schootman M, Evanoff BA, Perlmutter JS, Racette BA. Neurologist care in Parkinson disease: a utilization, outcomes, and survival study. Neurology 2011;77:851-7.

51.   Okun MS. Neurologist Care Reduces Hospitalizations in Parkinson's Disease. What's Hot in Parkinson's Disease. http://www.parkinson.org2012 December.

52.   Oguh O, Kwasny M, Carter J, Stell B, Simuni T. Caregiver strain in Parkinson's disease: national Parkinson Foundation Quality Initiative study. Parkinsonism & related disorders 2013;19:975-9.

53.   Carter JH, Stewart BJ, Archbold PG, et al. Living with a person who has Parkinson's disease: the spouse's perspective by stage of disease. Parkinson's Study Group. Movement disorders : official journal of the Movement Disorder Society 1998;13:20-8.

54.   Carter JH, Stewart BJ, Lyons KS, Archbold PG. Do motor and nonmotor symptoms in PD patients predict caregiver strain and depression? Movement disorders : official journal of the Movement Disorder Society 2008;23:1211-6.

55.   Fahn S, Poewe W. Levodopa: 50 years of a revolutionary drug for Parkinson disease. Movement disorders : official journal of the Movement Disorder Society 2015;30:1-3.

56.   LeWitt PA, Nelson MV, Berchou RC, et al. Controlled-release carbidopa/levodopa (Sinemet 50/200 CR4): clinical and pharmacokinetic studies. Neurology 1989;39:45-53; discussion 9.

57.   LeWitt PA. Clinical studies with and pharmacokinetic considerations of sustained-release levodopa. Neurology 1992;42:29-32; discussion 57-60.

58.   Parcopa: a rapidly dissolving formulation of carbidopa/levodopa. The Medical letter on drugs and therapeutics 2005;47:12.

59.   Hauser RA. IPX066: a novel carbidopa-levodopa extended-release formulation. Expert review of neurotherapeutics 2012;12:133-40.

60.   Hauser RA, Hsu A, Kell S, et al. Extended-release carbidopa-levodopa (IPX066) compared with immediate-release carbidopa-levodopa in patients with Parkinson's disease and motor fluctuations: a phase 3 randomised, double-blind trial. The Lancet Neurology 2013;12:346-56.

61.   Okun MS. Tips for Parkinson's Disease Patients Switching from Sinemet or Madopar to Rytary (IPX066). What's Hot in Parkinson's Disease. http://www.parkinson.org2015 May.

62.   Go CL, Rosales RL, Schmidt P, Lyons KE, Pahwa R, Okun MS. Generic versus branded pharmacotherapy in Parkinson's disease: does it matter? A review. Parkinsonism & related disorders 2011;17:308-12.

63.   Brodell DW, Stanford NT, Jacobson CE, Schmidt P, Okun MS. Carbidopa/levodopa dose elevation and safety concerns in Parkinson's patients: a cross-sectional and cohort design. BMJ open 2012;2.

64.   Okun MS. Parkinson's disease patients cannot get their dopamine replacement: the 8-Sinemet limit. Movement disorders : official journal of the Movement Disorder Society 2012;27:461-2.

65.   Okun MS. Pill Color, Generic Medications and Insurance Issues: Important Medication-Related Tips for the Parkinson's Disease Patient. What's Hot in Parkinson's Disease. http://www.parkinson.org2012 February.

66.   Antonini A, Cilia R. Behavioural adverse effects of dopaminergic treatments in Parkinson's disease: incidence, neurobiological basis, management and prevention. Drug safety 2009;32:475-88.

67.   Evans AH, Strafella AP, Weintraub D, Stacy M. Impulsive and compulsive behaviors in Parkinson's disease. Movement disorders : official journal of the Movement Disorder Society 2009;24:1561-70.

68.   Giugni JC, Okun MS. Treatment of advanced Parkinson's disease. Current opinion in neurology 2014;27:450-60.

69.   Limotai N, Oyama G, Go C, et al. Addiction-like manifestations and Parkinson's disease: a large single center 9-year experience. The International journal of neuroscience 2012;122:145-53.

70.   Dewey RB, 2nd, Reimold SC, O'Suilleabhain PE. Cardiac valve regurgitation with pergolide compared with nonergot agonists in Parkinson disease. Archives of neurology 2007;64:377-80.

71.   Parkinson Study G. Pramipexole vs levodopa as initial treatment for Parkinson disease: A randomized controlled trial. Parkinson Study Group. Jama 2000;284:1931-8.

72.   Rascol O, Brooks DJ, Korczyn AD, De Deyn PP, Clarke CE, Lang AE. A five-year study of the incidence of dyskinesia in patients with early Parkinson's disease who were treated with ropinirole or levodopa. The New England journal of medicine 2000;342:1484-91.

73.   Weintraub D, Siderowf AD, Potenza MN, et al. Association of dopamine agonist use with impulse control disorders in Parkinson disease. Archives of neurology 2006;63:969-73.

74.   Garcia-Ruiz PJ, Martinez Castrillo JC, Alonso-Canovas A, et al. Impulse control disorder in patients with Parkinson's disease under dopamine agonist therapy: a multicentre study. Journal of neurology, neurosurgery, and psychiatry 2014;85:840-4.

75.   Okun MS, Siderowf A, Nutt JG, et al. Piloting the NPF data-driven quality improvement initiative. Parkinsonism & related disorders 2010;16:517-21.

76.   Samuel M, Rodriguez-Oroz M, Antonini A, et al. Management of impulse control disorders in Parkinson's disease: Controversies and future approaches. Movement disorders : official journal of the Movement Disorder Society 2015;30:150-9.

77.   Henriksen T. Clinical insights into use of apomorphine in Parkinson's disease: tools for clinicians. Neurodegenerative disease management 2014;4:271-82.

78.   Wenzel K, Homann CN, Fabbrini G, Colosimo C. The role of subcutaneous infusion of apomorphine in Parkinson's disease. Expert review of neurotherapeutics 2014;14:833-43.

79.   Brunerova L, Potockova J, Horacek J, Koprivova H, Rehula M, Andel M. Sublingual apomorphine as a neuroendocrine probe. Psychiatry research 2012;198:297-9.

80.   Okun MS. Given the recent FDA announcement about Mirapex (pramipexole), should I be worried about dopamine agonists? What's Hot in Parkinson's Disease. http://www.parkinson.org2012 October.

81.   Okun MS. The Importance of a Monitoring Strategy When Prescribing Dopamine Agonists: Lessons from the National Parkinson Foundation Data. What's Hot in Parkinson's Disease. http://www.parkinson.org2014 November.

82.   Marsala SZ, Gioulis M, Ceravolo R, Tinazzi M. A systematic review of catechol-0-methyltransferase inhibitors: efficacy and safety in clinical practice. Clinical neuropharmacology 2012;35:185-90.

83.   Stocchi F, Rascol O, Kieburtz K, et al. Initiating levodopa/carbidopa therapy with and without entacapone in early Parkinson disease: the STRIDE-PD study. Annals of neurology 2010;68:18-27.

84.   Ferreira JJ, Rocha JF, Falcao A, et al. Effect of opicapone on levodopa pharmacokinetics, catechol-O-methyltransferase activity and motor fluctuations in patients with Parkinson's disease. European journal of neurology : the official journal of the European Federation of Neurological Societies 2015;22:815-e56.

85.   Olanow CW, Rascol O. The delayed-start study in Parkinson disease: can't satisfy everyone. Neurology 2010;74:1149-50.

86.   Olanow CW, Rascol O, Hauser R, et al. A double-blind, delayed-start trial of rasagiline in Parkinson's disease. The New England journal of medicine 2009;361:1268-78.

87.　　Giladi N, McDermott MP, Fahn S, et al. Freezing of gait in PD: prospective assessment in the DATATOP cohort. Neurology 2001;56:1712-21.

88.　　Borgohain R, Szasz J, Stanzione P, et al. Two-year, randomized, controlled study of safinamide as add-on to levodopa in mid to late Parkinson's disease. Movement disorders : official journal of the Movement Disorder Society 2014;29:1273-80.

89.　　Kurlan R. "Levodopa phobia": a new iatrogenic cause of disability in Parkinson disease. Neurology 2005;64:923-4.

90.　　Bertoni JM, Arlette JP, Fernandez HH, et al. Increased melanoma risk in Parkinson disease: a prospective clinicopathological study. Archives of neurology 2010;67:347-52.

91.　　Okun MS. When Should I Start a Medicine for Parkinson's Disease. What's Hot in Parkinson's Disease. http://www.parkinson.org2013 January.

92.　　Parkkinen L, O'Sullivan SS, Kuoppamaki M, et al. Does levodopa accelerate the pathologic process in Parkinson disease brain? Neurology 2011;77:1420-6.

93.　　Fahn S. Parkinson disease, the effect of levodopa, and the ELLDOPA trial. Earlier vs Later L-DOPA. Archives of neurology 1999;56:529-35.

94.　　Fahn S, Parkinson Study G. Does levodopa slow or hasten the rate of progression of Parkinson's disease? Journal of neurology 2005;252 Suppl 4:IV37-IV42.

95.　　Lang AE, Marras C. Initiating dopaminergic treatment in Parkinson's disease. Lancet 2014;384:1164-6.

96.　　Group PDMC, Gray R, Ives N, et al. Long-term effectiveness of dopamine agonists and monoamine oxidase B inhibitors compared with levodopa as initial treatment for Parkinson's disease (PD MED): a large, open-label, pragmatic randomised trial. Lancet 2014;384:1196-205.

97.　　Okun MS. The End for Levodopa Phobia: New Study Shows Sinemet is a Safe Initial Therapy for Treatment of Parkinson's Disease. What's Hot in Parkinson's Disease. http://www.parkinson.org2014 July.

98.　　Koppel BS, Brust JC, Fife T, et al. Systematic review: efficacy and safety of medical marijuana in selected neurologic disorders: report of the Guideline Development Subcommittee of the American Academy of Neurology. Neurology 2014;82:1556-63.

99.   Venderova K, Ruzicka E, Vorisek V, Visnovsky P. Survey on cannabis use in Parkinson's disease: subjective improvement of motor symptoms. Movement disorders : official journal of the Movement Disorder Society 2004;19:1102-6.

100.   Volkow ND, Compton WM, Weiss SR. Adverse health effects of marijuana use. The New England journal of medicine 2014;371:879.

101.   Kluger B, Triolo P, Jones W, Jankovic J. The therapeutic potential of cannabinoids for movement disorders. Movement disorders : official journal of the Movement Disorder Society 2015;30:313-27.

102.   Okun MS. Everything You Need to Know About Medical Marijuana and Parkinson's Disease. What's Hot in Parkinson's Disease. http://www.parkinson.org2014 August.

103.   Fernandez HH, Trieschmann ME, Okun MS. Rebound psychosis: effect of discontinuation of antipsychotics in Parkinson's disease. Movement disorders : official journal of the Movement Disorder Society 2005;20:104-5.

104.   Hack N, Fayad SM, Monari EH, et al. An eight-year clinic experience with clozapine use in a Parkinson's disease clinic setting. PloS one 2014;9:e91545.

105.   Wint DP, Okun MS, Fernandez HH. Psychosis in Parkinson's disease. Journal of geriatric psychiatry and neurology 2004;17:127-36.

106.   Baik HM, Choe BY, Son BC, et al. Proton MR spectroscopic changes in Parkinson's diseases after thalamotomy. European journal of radiology 2003;47:179-87.

107.   Borek LL, Friedman JH. Treating psychosis in movement disorder patients: a review. Expert opinion on pharmacotherapy 2014;15:1553-64.

108.   Broadstock M, Ballard C, Corbett A. Novel pharmaceuticals in the treatment of psychosis in Parkinson's disease. Expert review of clinical pharmacology 2014;7:779-86.

109.   Cummings J, Isaacson S, Mills R, et al. Pimavanserin for patients with Parkinson's disease psychosis: a randomised, placebo-controlled phase 3 trial. Lancet 2014;383:533-40.

110.   Friedman JH. Pimavanserin for the treatment of Parkinson's disease psychosis. Expert opinion on pharmacotherapy 2013;14:1969-75.

111.   Kingwell K. Parkinson disease: Pimavanserin could be useful for treating psychosis in Parkinson disease. Nature reviews Neurology 2013;9:658.

112.   Meltzer HY, Roth BL. Lorcaserin and pimavanserin: emerging selectivity of serotonin receptor subtype-targeted drugs. The Journal of clinical investigation 2013;123:4986-91.

113.   Okun MS. Pimavanserin and the Hope for a Better Drug for Hallucinations and Psychosis in Parkinson's Disease. What's Hot in Parkinson's Disease. http://www.parkinson.org2013 November.

114.   Videnovic A, Breen DP, Barker RA, Zee PC. The central clock in patients with Parkinson disease--reply. JAMA neurology 2014;71:1456-7.

115.   Videnovic A, Lazar AS, Barker RA, Overeem S. 'The clocks that time us'--circadian rhythms in neurodegenerative disorders. Nature reviews Neurology 2014;10:683-93.

116.   Okun MS. Is light therapy a potential treatment modality in Parkinson's disease? What's Hot in Parkinson's Disease. http://www.parkinson.org2015 May.

117.   Gras-Miralles B, Cremonini F. A critical appraisal of lubiprostone in the treatment of chronic constipation in the elderly. Clinical interventions in aging 2013;8:191-200.

118.   Ondo WG, Kenney C, Sullivan K, et al. Placebo-controlled trial of lubiprostone for constipation associated with Parkinson disease. Neurology 2012;78:1650-4.

119.   Herzberg L. An essay on the shaking palsy: reviews and notes on the journals in which they appeared. Movement disorders : official journal of the Movement Disorder Society 1990;5:162-6.

120.   Camilleri M, Acosta A. Emerging treatments in Neurogastroenterology: relamorelin: a novel gastrocolokinetic synthetic ghrelin agonist. Neurogastroenterology and motility : the official journal of the European Gastrointestinal Motility Society 2015;27:324-32.

121.   Mozaffari S, Didari T, Nikfar S, Abdollahi M. Phase II drugs under clinical investigation for the treatment of chronic constipation. Expert opinion on investigational drugs 2014;23:1485-97.

122.   Shin A, Wo JM. Therapeutic applications of ghrelin agonists in the treatment of gastroparesis. Current gastroenterology reports 2015;17:430.

123.   Okun MS. A New Treatment for Parkinson's Disease-Related Constipation. What's Hot in Parkinson's Disease. http://www.parkinson.org2012 June.

124.   Ha AD, Brown CH, York MK, Jankovic J. The prevalence of symptomatic orthostatic hypotension in patients with Parkinson's disease and atypical parkinsonism. Parkinsonism & related disorders 2011;17:625-8.

125.   Jankovic J, Gilden JL, Hiner BC, et al. Neurogenic orthostatic hypotension: a double-blind, placebo-controlled study with midodrine. The American journal of medicine 1993;95:38-48.

126.   Mostile G, Jankovic J. Treatment of dysautonomia associated with Parkinson's disease. Parkinsonism & related disorders 2009;15 Suppl 3:S224-32.

127.   Biaggioni I. New developments in the management of neurogenic orthostatic hypotension. Current cardiology reports 2014;16:542.

128.   Isaacson SH, Skettini J. Neurogenic orthostatic hypotension in Parkinson's disease: evaluation, management, and emerging role of droxidopa. Vascular health and risk management 2014;10:169-76.

129.   Wu CK, Hohler AD. Management of orthostatic hypotension in patients with Parkinson's disease. Practical neurology 2015;15:100-4.

130.   Biaggioni I, Freeman R, Mathias CJ, et al. Randomized withdrawal study of patients with symptomatic neurogenic orthostatic hypotension responsive to droxidopa. Hypertension 2015;65:101-7.

131.   Hauser RA, Hewitt LA, Isaacson S. Droxidopa in patients with neurogenic orthostatic hypotension associated with Parkinson's disease (NOH306A). Journal of Parkinson's disease 2014;4:57-65.

132.   Hauser RA, Isaacson S, Lisk JP, Hewitt LA, Rowse G. Droxidopa for the Short-Term Treatment of Symptomatic Neurogenic Orthostatic Hypotension in Parkinson's Disease (nOH306B). Movement disorders : official journal of the Movement Disorder Society 2015;30:646-54.

133.   Kaufmann H, Freeman R, Biaggioni I, et al. Droxidopa for neurogenic orthostatic hypotension: a randomized, placebo-controlled, phase 3 trial. Neurology 2014;83:328-35.

134.   Okun MS. Could Northera (Droxidopa) Be an Alternative Treatment for Low Blood Pressure and Passing Out Symptoms in Parkinson's Disease? What's Hot in Parkinson's Disease. http://www.parkinson.org2015 May.

135.   Low V, Ben-Shlomo Y, Coward E, Fletcher S, Walker R, Clarke CE. Measuring the burden and mortality of hospitalisation in Parkinson's disease:

A cross-sectional analysis of the English Hospital Episodes Statistics database 2009-2013. Parkinsonism & related disorders 2015.

136.   Skelly R, Brown L, Fakis A, et al. Does a specialist unit improve outcomes for hospitalized patients with Parkinson's disease? Parkinsonism & related disorders 2014;20:1242-7.

137.   Skelly R, Brown L, Fakis A, Walker R. Hospitalization in Parkinson's disease: a survey of UK neurologists, geriatricians and Parkinson's disease nurse specialists. Parkinsonism & related disorders 2015;21:277-81.

138.   Aminoff MJ, Christine CW, Friedman JH, et al. Management of the hospitalized patient with Parkinson's disease: current state of the field and need for guidelines. Parkinsonism & related disorders 2011;17:139-45.

139.   Hassan A, Wu SS, Schmidt P, et al. High rates and the risk factors for emergency room visits and hospitalization in Parkinson's disease. Parkinsonism & related disorders 2013;19:949-54.

140.   Chou KL, Zamudio J, Schmidt P, et al. Hospitalization in Parkinson disease: a survey of National Parkinson Foundation Centers. Parkinsonism & related disorders 2011;17:440-5.

141.   Shahgholi L, De Jesus, S., Wu, S., Pei, Q., Hassan, A., Schmidt, P., Okun, M.S. The Profile of the Hospitalized and Re-Hospitalized Parkinson Disease Patient: 5 Year Data from the National Parkinson Foundation American Academy of Neurology Washington DC2015.

142.   Martinez-Ramirez D, Giugni JC, Little CS, et al. Missing dosages and neuroleptic usage may prolong length of stay in hospitalized Parkinson's disease patients. PloS one 2015;10:e0124356.

143.   Okun MS. A Critical Reappraisal of the Worst Drugs in Parkinson's Disease. What's Hot in Parkinson's Disease. http://www.parkinson.org2011 January.

144.   Olanow CW, Obeso J. Profile of Mahlon DeLong and Alim Benabid, 2014 Lasker-DeBakey Medical Research awardees. Proceedings of the National Academy of Sciences of the United States of America 2014;111:17693-5.

145.   DeLong MR, Benabid AL. Discovery of high-frequency deep brain stimulation for treatment of Parkinson disease: 2014 Lasker Award. Jama 2014;312:1093-4.

146.   Benabid AL. Neuroscience: spotlight on deep-brain stimulation. Nature 2015;519:299-300.

147.   Benabid AL. Lasker Award winner Alim Louis Benabid. Nature medicine 2014;20:1121-3.

148.   Okun MS. Deep-brain stimulation--entering the era of human neural-network modulation. The New England journal of medicine 2014;371:1369-73.

149.   Okun MS, Oyama G. Mechanism of action for deep brain stimulation and electrical neuro-network modulation (ENM). Rinsho shinkeigaku = Clinical neurology 2013;53:691-4.

150.   McIntyre CC, Hahn PJ. Network perspectives on the mechanisms of deep brain stimulation. Neurobiology of disease 2010;38:329-37.

151.   McIntyre CC, Foutz TJ. Computational modeling of deep brain stimulation. Handbook of clinical neurology 2013;116:55-61.

152.   Birdno MJ, Grill WM. Mechanisms of deep brain stimulation in movement disorders as revealed by changes in stimulus frequency. Neurotherapeutics : the journal of the American Society for Experimental NeuroTherapeutics 2008;5:14-25.

153.   Zhang TC, Grill WM. Modeling deep brain stimulation: point source approximation versus realistic representation of the electrode. Journal of neural engineering 2010;7:066009.

154.   de Hemptinne C, Swann NC, Ostrem JL, et al. Therapeutic deep brain stimulation reduces cortical phase-amplitude coupling in Parkinson's disease. Nature neuroscience 2015;18:779-86.

155.   Vedam-Mai V, Gardner B, Okun MS, et al. Increased precursor cell proliferation after deep brain stimulation for Parkinson's disease: a human study. PloS one 2014;9:e88770.

156.   Vedam-Mai V, Krock N, Ullman M, et al. The national DBS brain tissue network pilot study: need for more tissue and more standardization. Cell and tissue banking 2011;12:219-31.

157.   Wang S, Okun MS, Suslov O, et al. Neurogenic potential of progenitor cells isolated from postmortem human Parkinsonian brains. Brain research 2012;1464:61-72.

158.   Okun MS, Fernandez HH, Pedraza O, et al. Development and initial validation of a screening tool for Parkinson disease surgical candidates. Neurology 2004;63:161-3.

159.   Okun MS, Foote KD. Parkinson's disease DBS: what, when, who and why? The time has come to tailor DBS targets. Expert review of neurotherapeutics 2010;10:1847-57.

160.   Weaver FM, Follett K, Stern M, et al. Bilateral deep brain stimulation vs best medical therapy for patients with advanced Parkinson disease: a randomized controlled trial. Jama 2009;301:63-73.

161.   Weaver FM, Follett KA, Stern M, et al. Randomized trial of deep brain stimulation for Parkinson disease: thirty-six-month outcomes. Neurology 2012;79:55-65.

162.   Follett KA, Weaver FM, Stern M, et al. Pallidal versus subthalamic deep-brain stimulation for Parkinson's disease. The New England journal of medicine 2010;362:2077-91.

163.   Williams NR, Foote KD, Okun MS. STN vs. GPi Deep Brain Stimulation: Translating the Rematch into Clinical Practice. Movement disorders clinical practice 2014;1:24-35.

164.   Okun MS, Foote KD. Subthalamic nucleus vs globus pallidus interna deep brain stimulation, the rematch: will pallidal deep brain stimulation make a triumphant return? Archives of neurology 2005;62:533-6.

165.   Tagliati M. Turning tables: should GPi become the preferred DBS target for Parkinson disease? Neurology 2012;79:19-20.

166.   Katz M, Luciano MS, Carlson K, et al. Differential effects of deep brain stimulation target on motor subtypes in Parkinson's disease. Annals of neurology 2015;77:710-9.

167.   Okun MS. Time to Consider GPi DBS for Parkinson's Disease: A Shift in the Practice of Patient Selection for DBS. What's Hot in Parkinson's Disease. http://www.parkinson.org2012 July.

168.   Schuepbach WM, Rau J, Knudsen K, et al. Neurostimulation for Parkinson's disease with early motor complications. The New England journal of medicine 2013;368:610-22.

169.   Charles D, Konrad PE, Davis TL, Neimat JS, Hacker ML, Finder SG. Deep brain stimulation in early stage Parkinson's disease. Parkinsonism & related disorders 2015;21:347-8.

170.   Barbe MT, Maarouf M, Alesch F, Timmermann L. Multiple source current steering--a novel deep brain stimulation concept for customized programming in a Parkinson's disease patient. Parkinsonism & related disorders 2014;20:471-3.

171.   Pollo C, Kaelin-Lang A, Oertel MF, et al. Directional deep brain stimulation: an intraoperative double-blind pilot study. Brain : a journal of neurology 2014;137:2015-26.

172.   Toader E, Decre MM, Martens HC. Steering deep brain stimulation fields using a high resolution electrode array. Conference proceedings : Annual International Conference of the IEEE Engineering in Medicine and Biology Society IEEE Engineering in Medicine and Biology Society Annual Conference 2010;2010:2061-4.

173.   Martens HC, Toader E, Decre MM, et al. Spatial steering of deep brain stimulation volumes using a novel lead design. Clinical neurophysiology : official journal of the International Federation of Clinical Neurophysiology 2011;122:558-66.

174.   Gunduz A, Morita H, Rossi PJ, et al. Proceedings of the Second Annual Deep Brain Stimulation Think Tank: What's in the Pipeline. The International journal of neuroscience 2014:1-31.

175.   Okun MS, Foote KD, Wu SS, et al. A trial of scheduled deep brain stimulation for Tourette syndrome: moving away from continuous deep brain stimulation paradigms. JAMA neurology 2013;70:85-94.

176.   Maling N, Hashemiyoon R, Foote KD, Okun MS, Sanchez JC. Increased thalamic gamma band activity correlates with symptom relief following deep brain stimulation in humans with Tourette's syndrome. PloS one 2012;7:e44215.

177.   Almeida L, Martinez-Ramirez D, Rossi PJ, Peng Z, Gunduz A, Okun MS. Chasing tics in the human brain: development of open, scheduled and closed loop responsive approaches to deep brain stimulation for tourette syndrome. Journal of clinical neurology 2015;11:122-31.

178.   Okun MS. Deep Brain Stimulation for Parkinson's Disease: NPF Congratulates Mahlon DeLong and Alim-Louis Benabid and Looks to a Bright Future in Human Neural-Network Modulation. What's Hot in Parkinson's Disease. http://www.parkinson.org2014 September.

179.   Olanow CW, Kieburtz K, Odin P, et al. Continuous intrajejunal infusion of levodopa-carbidopa intestinal gel for patients with advanced Parkinson's disease: a randomised, controlled, double-blind, double-dummy study. The Lancet Neurology 2014;13:141-9.

180.   Guthikonda LN, Lyons KE, Pahwa R. Continuous infusion of levodopa-carbidopa intestinal gel in Parkinson's disease. Journal of comparative effectiveness research 2014;3:331-3.

181.   Okun MS. Everything a Parkinson's Disease Patient Needs to Know About the New Dopamine Pump. What's Hot in Parkinson's Disease. http://www.parkinson.org2015 March.

182.   Senek M, Nyholm D. Continuous drug delivery in Parkinson's disease. CNS drugs 2014;28:19-27.

183.   Andres RH, Meyer M, Ducray AD, Widmer HR. Restorative neuroscience: concepts and perspectives. Swiss Med Wkly 2008;138:155-72.

184.   Arias-Carrion O, Freundlieb N, Oertel WH, Hoglinger GU. Adult neurogenesis and Parkinson's disease. CNS Neurol Disord Drug Targets 2007;6:326-35.

185.   Park DH, Borlongan CV, Eve DJ, Sanberg PR. The emerging field of cell and tissue engineering. Med Sci Monit 2008;14:RA206-20.

186.   Steindler DA. Stem cells, regenerative medicine, and animal models of disease. Ilar J 2007;48:323-38.

187.   Svendsen C. Stem cells and Parkinson's disease: toward a treatment, not a cure. Cell Stem Cell 2008;2:412-3.

188.   Trzaska KA, Rameshwar P. Current advances in the treatment of Parkinson's disease with stem cells. Curr Neurovasc Res 2007;4:99-109.

189.   Oh SK, Choo AB. Human embryonic stem cell technology: large scale cell amplification and differentiation. Cytotechnology 2006;50:181-90.

190.   McKay R, Kittappa R. Will stem cell biology generate new therapies for Parkinson's disease? Neuron 2008;58:659-61.

191. Deuschl G. [Therapy of Parkinson's disease 2008]. MMW Fortschr Med 2008;150 Suppl 2:60-3.

192. Alexander GE, Crutcher MD, DeLong MR. Basal ganglia-thalamocortical circuits: parallel substrates for motor, oculomotor, "prefrontal" and "limbic" functions. Prog Brain Res 1990;85:119-46.

193. Alexander GE, DeLong MR, Strick PL. Parallel organization of functionally segregated circuits linking basal ganglia and cortex. Annu Rev Neurosci 1986;9:357-81.

194. Weiner WJ. There is no Parkinson disease. Arch Neurol 2008;65:705-8.

195. Saporta MA, Grskovic M, Dimos JT. Induced pluripotent stem cells in the study of neurological diseases. Stem cell research & therapy 2011;2:37.

196. Sanchez-Danes A, Richaud-Patin Y, Carballo-Carbajal I, et al. Disease-specific phenotypes in dopamine neurons from human iPS-based models of genetic and sporadic Parkinson's disease. EMBO molecular medicine 2012;4:380-95.

197. Ole I. Opportunities for neurorestorative therapies in PD using iPS and stem cells. Rinsho shinkeigaku = Clinical neurology 2010;50:891.

198. Imamura K, Inoue H. Research on neurodegenerative diseases using induced pluripotent stem cells. Psychogeriatrics : the official journal of the Japanese Psychogeriatric Society 2012;12:115-9.

199. Barker RA, de Beaufort I. Scientific and ethical issues related to stem cell research and interventions in neurodegenerative disorders of the brain. Progress in neurobiology 2013;110:63-73.

200. Okun MS. New iPS Stem Cells for PD: What Does it Mean? What's Hot in Parkinson's Disease. http://www.parkinson.org2010 March.

201. Okun MS. Placing Stem Cells in Animal Models of Parkinson's Disease: Another Important Step. What's Hot in Parkinson's Disease. http://www.parkinson.org2011 December.

202. Blesa J. Parkinson's disease: "Braak" to the future. Movement disorders : official journal of the Movement Disorder Society 2013;28:1209.

203. Visanji NP, Brooks PL, Hazrati LN, Lang AE. The prion hypothesis in Parkinson's disease: Braak to the future. Acta neuropathologica communications 2013;1:2.

204.	Prusiner SB. Creutzfeldt-Jakob disease and scrapie prions. Alzheimer disease and associated disorders 1989;3:52-78.

205.	Olanow CW, Prusiner SB. Is Parkinson's disease a prion disorder? Proceedings of the National Academy of Sciences of the United States of America 2009;106:12571-2.

206.	Brundin P, Kordower JH. Neuropathology in transplants in Parkinson's disease: implications for disease pathogenesis and the future of cell therapy. Progress in brain research 2012;200:221-41.

207.	Braak H, Rub U, Jansen Steur EN, Del Tredici K, de Vos RA. Cognitive status correlates with neuropathologic stage in Parkinson disease. Neurology 2005;64:1404-10.

208.	Braak H, Rub U, Del Tredici K. Cognitive decline correlates with neuropathological stage in Parkinson's disease. Journal of the neurological sciences 2006;248:255-8.

209.	Braak H, Muller CM, Rub U, et al. Pathology associated with sporadic Parkinson's disease--where does it end? Journal of neural transmission Supplementum 2006:89-97.

210.	Braak H, Del Tredici K, Rub U, de Vos RA, Jansen Steur EN, Braak E. Staging of brain pathology related to sporadic Parkinson's disease. Neurobiology of aging 2003;24:197-211.

211.	Braak H, Del Tredici K, Bratzke H, Hamm-Clement J, Sandmann-Keil D, Rub U. Staging of the intracerebral inclusion body pathology associated with idiopathic Parkinson's disease (preclinical and clinical stages). Journal of neurology 2002;249 Suppl 3:III/1-5.

212.	Ugen KE, Lin X, Bai G, et al. Evaluation of an alpha synuclein sensitized dendritic cell based vaccine in a transgenic mouse model of Parkinson disease. Human vaccines & immunotherapeutics 2015;11:922-30.

213.	Ghochikyan A, Petrushina I, Davtyan H, et al. Immunogenicity of epitope vaccines targeting different B cell antigenic determinants of human alpha-synuclein: feasibility study. Neuroscience letters 2014;560:86-91.

214.	Guerrero-Munoz MJ, Castillo-Carranza DL, Kayed R. Therapeutic approaches against common structural features of toxic oligomers shared by multiple amyloidogenic proteins. Biochemical pharmacology 2014;88:468-78.

215. Rohn TT. Targeting alpha-synuclein for the treatment of Parkinson's disease. CNS & neurological disorders drug targets 2012;11:174-9.

216. Tran HT, Chung CH, Iba M, et al. Alpha-synuclein immunotherapy blocks uptake and templated propagation of misfolded alpha-synuclein and neurodegeneration. Cell reports 2014;7:2054-65.

217. Ha D, Stone DK, Mosley RL, Gendelman HE. Immunization strategies for Parkinson's disease. Parkinsonism & related disorders 2012;18 Suppl 1:S218-21.

218. Okun MS. Two New Therapies for Parkinson's Disease Patients to get Excited About: Vaccines and Monoclonal Antibodies. What's Hot in Parkinson's Disease. http://www.parkinson.org2014 December.

219. Bartus RT, Baumann TL, Siffert J, et al. Safety/feasibility of targeting the substantia nigra with AAV2-neurturin in Parkinson patients. Neurology 2013;80:1698-701.

220. Hickey P, Stacy M. AAV2-neurturin (CERE-120) for Parkinson's disease. Expert opinion on biological therapy 2013;13:137-45.

221. Kordower JH, Bjorklund A. Trophic factor gene therapy for Parkinson's disease. Movement disorders : official journal of the Movement Disorder Society 2013;28:96-109.

222. Christine CW, Starr PA, Larson PS, et al. Safety and tolerability of putaminal AADC gene therapy for Parkinson disease. Neurology 2009;73:1662-9.

223. Mittermeyer G, Christine CW, Rosenbluth KH, et al. Long-term evaluation of a phase 1 study of AADC gene therapy for Parkinson's disease. Human gene therapy 2012;23:377-81.

224. LeWitt PA, Rezai AR, Leehey MA, et al. AAV2-GAD gene therapy for advanced Parkinson's disease: a double-blind, sham-surgery controlled, randomised trial. The Lancet Neurology 2011;10:309-19.

225. Palfi S, Gurruchaga JM, Ralph GS, et al. Long-term safety and tolerability of ProSavin, a lentiviral vector-based gene therapy for Parkinson's disease: a dose escalation, open-label, phase 1/2 trial. Lancet 2014;383:1138-46.

226. Okun MS. Update on Gene Therapy for Parkinson's Disease. What's Hot in Parkinson's Disease. http://www.parkinson.org2008 November.

227.   Okun MS. Opening the Door to Gene Therapy in Parkinson's Disease: The Need for Refinement of the Technology and Approach. What's Hot in Parkinson's Disease: http://www.parkinson.org; 2011 April.

228.   Freeze BS, Kravitz AV, Hammack N, Berke JD, Kreitzer AC. Control of basal ganglia output by direct and indirect pathway projection neurons. The Journal of neuroscience : the official journal of the Society for Neuroscience 2013;33:18531-9.

229.   Kravitz AV, Kreitzer AC. Optogenetic manipulation of neural circuitry in vivo. Current opinion in neurobiology 2011;21:433-9.

230.   Kravitz AV, Owen SF, Kreitzer AC. Optogenetic identification of striatal projection neuron subtypes during in vivo recordings. Brain research 2013;1511:21-32.

231.   Bass CE, Grinevich VP, Gioia D, et al. Optogenetic stimulation of VTA dopamine neurons reveals that tonic but not phasic patterns of dopamine transmission reduce ethanol self-administration. Frontiers in behavioral neuroscience 2013;7:173.

232.   Bass CE, Grinevich VP, Kulikova AD, Bonin KD, Budygin EA. Terminal effects of optogenetic stimulation on dopamine dynamics in rat striatum. Journal of neuroscience methods 2013;214:149-55.

233.   Bass CE, Grinevich VP, Vance ZB, Sullivan RP, Bonin KD, Budygin EA. Optogenetic control of striatal dopamine release in rats. Journal of neurochemistry 2010;114:1344-52.

234.   Okun MS. Shining a Light on Parkinson's Disease: Optogenetics Has a Bright Future in Research. What's Hot in Parkinson's Disease. http://www.parkinson.org2010 August.

3/17

41431852R00088

Made in the USA
Middletown, DE
11 March 2017